OXFORD MEDICAL PUBLICATIONS

DEAFNESS

THE FACTS

ALSO PUBLISHED BY OXFORD UNIVERSITY PRESS

DEAFNESS

THE FACTS

ANDREW P. FREELAND

Consultant ENT Surgeon,
Radcliffe Infirmary, Oxford;
Clinical Lecturer,
University of Oxford

OXFORD NEW YORK TOKYO
OXFORD UNIVERSITY PRESS
1989

Oxford University Press, Walton Street, Oxford OX2 6DP
Oxford New York Toronto
Delhi Bombay Calcutta Madras Karachi
Petaling Jaya Singapore Hong Kong Tokyo
Nairobi Dar es Salaam Cape Town
Melbourne Auckland
and associated companies in
Berlin Ibadan

Oxford is a trade mark of Oxford University Press

Published in the United States
by Oxford University Press, New York

British Library Cataloguing in Publication Data
Freeland, Andrew
Deafness.
1. Man. Deafness
I. Title
617.8
ISBN 0–19–261741–9
0–19–261796–6 (pbk.)

Library of Congress Cataloging in Publication Data
Freeland, Andrew.
Deafness : the facts / Andrew Freeland.
(Oxford medical publications)
Includes index.
1. Deafness. I. Title. II. Series.
RF290.F74   1989   617.8—dc19   88–26581
ISBN 0–19–261741–9
ISBN 0–19–261796–6 (pbk.)

Set by Footnote Graphics, Warminster, Wilts.
Printed in Great Britain by
Biddles Ltd, Guildford and King's Lynn

PREFACE AND ACKNOWLEDGEMENTS

Although there are a great many textbooks on ear disease and deafness, few are understandable by the general public. I hope this little book will provide a readable, up-to-date account of the problems of deafness for the lay person. The ear is a complex organ and doctors and other health workers are frequently accused of not adequately explaining disease processes to their patients. I hope these chapters will help to clarify the mysteries of hearing and lack of it to the patient, parent, relative, or anyone else interested in the subject. I am indebted, for many of the thoughts, to my patients from whom I have learnt so much.

I am grateful to the staff of Oxford University Press for their support. The help of Mrs Jane Jones, Senior Children's Hearing Therapist at the Radcliffe Infirmary, Oxford, has been invaluable. The special knowledge which comes from her expert handling and teaching of hearing-impaired children was most useful in the preparation of this book, particularly Chapters 6 and 7, which are concerned with the management of the deaf child. Thanks are also due to the audiology staff in the Radcliffe Infirmary for their advice on hearing tests and aids. Mr David Floyd of the Department of Medical Illustration at the John Radcliffe Hospital, Oxford prepared the photographs. Special thanks go to Miss Jo Dyer of the same department for her patience and skill in producing line drawings. Finally I am deeply indebted to my ex-secretary, Miss Christine Westwood, who has cheerfully spent her last university vacation typing and retyping the manuscript as well as correcting my English and spelling.

Oxford   A. P. F.
1988

CONTENTS

Contents

1

INTRODUCTION

'Deaf' is a common, everyday word that most people use to describe those who do not hear well and it is in this context that the word 'deafness' is used in this book; unless otherwise stated, it is not intended to mean total loss of hearing.

The problem of deafness is massive and is increasing as the human race lives longer. In the USA there are 30 million people with deafness, of whom 21 million are over the age of 65 years. In the UK seven million (one in six adults) are said to suffer from some degree of hearing loss and 70 per cent of these are over the age of 70. More than 1.5 million adults in the UK have been supplied with hearing aids and it is estimated that a further four million could benefit.

The handicaps of visual and hearing impairment are often compared and there is no doubt that blindness rates the highest degree of pity and sympathy. Yet, while blindness cuts people off from objects, deafness cuts people off from people. This results in social isolation, which surely deserves as much sympathy as blindness. Visual problems can usually be treated with spectacles which very successfully correct the problem. Hearing aids are not as socially acceptable as spectacles; nor are they as efficient at correcting the handicap. There is therefore a natural reluctance to wear them, leading to increasing withdrawal from the social scene. The deaf are often ignored, insulted, or considered dull witted. Many famous and eloquent people have been smitten by the handicap of deafness; Beethoven wrote: 'though endowed with a passionate and lively temperament and ever fond of the distractions offered by society, I was soon obliged to seclude myself and live in solitude'.

Since the industrial revolution, noise has reared its ugly head as a significant causative factor in hearing loss. The ageing process takes place naturally but noise, however apparently insignificant, contributes to this natural deterioration. Studies of some rural tribes not subjected to noise have shown significantly better hearing in their elderly populations than in equivalent populations in western urban society.

Most of us eventually develop some difficulty in hearing, particularly in noisy situations—for instance when holding a conversation in a pub or other social gathering. We all need to be better informed on the problem of hearing loss, on preventative measures such as noise protection, and on how to make the burden of deafness more tolerable. It is hoped that this book will go some way to achieving this goal.

WHAT OF THE FUTURE?

Modern, highly sophisticated microsurgery can restore the hearing in only a relatively small proportion of the huge number of people suffering from deafness. Prevention is the key to controlling any disease process. In recent years this has been demonstrated by the prevention of rubella (German measles) in pregnancy by widespread vaccination of non-immune teenage girls, by much improved baby care at birth, and by greater attention to childhood ear disease, which seems to be leading to fewer chronic problems in adults. Noise-protection programmes need urgently to be stepped up.

The future generation must be made more aware of the whole problem of deafness and encouraged to accept hearing aids as naturally as we do spectacles at present. Modern micro-electronics are rapidly improving and hopefully 'intelligent' hearing aids which can distinguish between background noise and speech will be developed. The role of cochlear implantation, which has attracted so much press speculation, will be discussed in the final chapter. It is indeed an exciting development, but of only limited application in those with total deafness. Fortunately, most hearing impaired people have at least remnants of hearing which can be significantly helped with a hearing aid.

Considering that hearing loss is probably the most common of all handicaps, the amount of money and time for research and development spent on it is pitifully small and this imbalance needs to be redressed to ensure that future generations of hearing-impaired have a better quality of life.

2

STRUCTURE AND FUNCTION

Let us consider first some of the amazing feats of the human ear; which even in our modern technological era put any man-made device years behind in comparison. The ear is not only highly sensitive, but also superbly selective. Its sensitivity is shown by the ability to respond to sounds ranging from the barely perceptible to those that can set the whole body vibrating, such as bomb blast or jet engine noise. Its selectivity is demonstrated, for example, by the ability to single out one person speaking in a room crowded with talking people, or that of the conductor of an orchestra to single out the one player who is not quite in tune or in time with the others. It has been calculated that at some sound frequencies the vibrations of the ear-drum are as small as one-billionth of a centimetre, or about one-tenth the diameter of a hydrogen atom, and those of the fine membrane in the inner ear, which transmits this stimulation to the nerve of hearing, are nearly a hundred times smaller.

Most people speak in the frequency range 500–3000 cycles per second, or Hertz (Hz) and it is in this range that the ear is most sensitive. At very low frequencies, such as 100 Hz, the ear is a thousand times less sensitive than at 1000 Hz. This is just as well because otherwise we would hear our own body vibrations. This fact can be demonstrated by placing a finger in each ear, which closes them to airborne sounds. A very low, irregular tone, which is produced by the contractions of the muscles of the arm and finger, can then be heard. It is interesting that the ear has just enough insensitivity to such low frequencies to avoid the disturbing effect of noises produced by muscles and bodily movements. At the high frequency end of the scale some children can hear frequencies as high as 40 000 Hz but with age the acuteness of perception of these sounds steadily drops. This process is perfectly natural and occurs with natural ageing of the rest of the body tissues.

STRUCTURE

Figure 1 shows the classical side view of the ear as seen in anatomical textbooks. It is useful since it divides the ear into the outer, middle, and inner parts. Each part has a specific function. The basic problem of hearing is that conduction of sound from the air to the brain is complicated by the fluid environment of the inner ear: sound waves are largely reflected off fluid (Fig. 2). To overcome this problem, the outer ear collects sound waves, and the middle ear converts this sound energy into a mechanical force; this is then

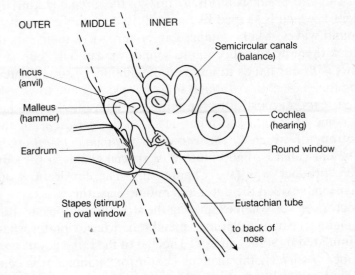

Fig. 1 Side view of ear showing division into outer, middle, and inner parts.

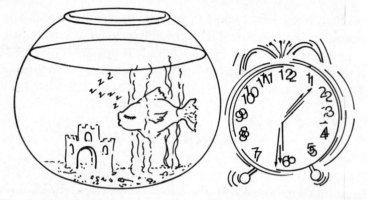

Fig. 2 Airborne sound does not easily penetrate fluid. The ear cleverly overcomes this problem when transmitting sound to the fluid-filled inner ear.

transmitted to the inner ear, converted to electrical energy, and sent via the *auditory nerve* to the brain. The outer and middle ear contain air, whereas the inner ear is in a fluid-filled space.

The *outer ear* comprises, firstly, the *pinna* (Latin for 'leaf'), which is shaped like a shell; its function is to collect sound waves. Many animals can either swivel their ears or prick them up to collect more sound; we can only 'cup' our ears with our hands to increase the amount of sound entering the ear-canal. Although some people are able to waggle their ears, in most of us the muscle responsible for this has become vestigial. The pinna leads to the *ear-canal*, at the bottom of which is the *ear-drum* (*tympanic membrane*). The ear-canal is slightly tortuous; special glands in the skin here produce wax (see Chapter 10). The ear-drum is the division between the outer and middle ears; this is as far as a doctor can see when examining the structure of the ear. It is a highly elastic, finely tuned membrane which vibrates when stimulated by sound energy. The first of the three middle ear bones (*ossicles*), the malleus (Latin for 'hammer'), is contained within its structure.

The *middle ear* is an air-containing space which contains

the three unusually shaped ossicles (Plate I): the *malleus* (*hammer*), *incus* (*anvil*), and *stapes* (*stirrup*). Sound waves received by the ear-drum cause it to vibrate, and this vibration passes in turn through the malleus, incus, and stapes, thus converting sound energy into mechanical energy. This energy is directed on to a membrane (the *oval window*) to which the stapes is connected, and which is 22 times smaller than the size of the ear-drum. The chain of ossicles thus acts much as a hydraulic press; it magnifies 22-fold the small pressures on the surface of the ear-drum and transmits them to the oval window. The oval window then sends the mechanical energy into the inner ear for conversion into electrical activity. One of the most important features of the middle ear is that it contains air, which is replenished via a tube (the *Eustachian tube*), which leads down from the middle ear through the skull to the back of the nose. As will be seen later, this tube is of great importance in such common conditions as glue ear (see Chapter 9). The tube is normally shut, but when we swallow the movement of the palate (roof of the mouth) opens it and allows more fresh air from the nose into the ear. This is the reason why passengers descending in an aeroplane are encouraged to chew sweets and to keep swallowing, since this automatically opens the Eustachian tube and allows the pressure in the middle ear to remain equal with that in the aircraft.

Just as the Eustachian tube connects the middle ear to the back of the nose, another opening in the roof of the middle ear connects it to the *mastoid bone*. The mastoid is felt as a hard bulge behind the ear. It has a hard outer shell but inside it is like a honeycomb of air-containing cells. It is variable in size and its function is not known. In the days before antibiotics it frequently became infected in children and surgical drainage was a common emergency procedure.

The ossicles are connected to each other by fluid-filled joints. Part of the reason for this is sound protection. When subjected to a very loud noise or loud blast the joints are able to dislocate partially, reducing the amount of energy being transmitted. This prevents harmful levels of vibration reaching the delicate inner ear.

The *inner ear* is an extraordinarily complicated mechanism and we do not yet fully understand exactly how the system works. It comprises a coiled structure called the *cochlea* (Latin for 'snail'). If it were straightened out, it would look like a U-tube (Fig. 3). One end is connected to the oval window; the other end is also in contact with another part of the middle ear through another membrane called the *round window*. The inner ear is fluid filled and

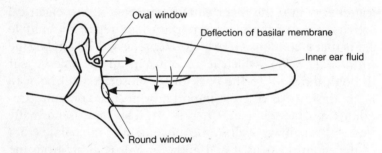

Fig. 3 Representation of the cochlear as a U-tube: sound energy enters the oval window causing a wave in the inner ear fluid. This displaces the basilar membrane at a point related to the specific frequency to be heard.

when the stapes moves a ripple is sent right through the fluid of the inner ear to the round window. This wave movement through the ear fluid is only possible because the round window, like the oval window, is elastic. At some point along the U-tube the ripple will have a maximum wave form; it is probable that this maximum wave represents the specific frequency of the sound being heard. The movement of the inner ear fluid deflects a thin membrane in the centre of this U-tube, called the *basilar membrane*. Delicate cells like tiny hairs balance on this membrane (the *organ of Corti*) and connect directly to a multitude of nerve endings, which join together to form the auditory (or acoustic) nerve. They transmit the sound to the brain.

Although we usually hear airborne sounds via the ear-canal and ear-drum, it is also possible to hear directly through the bone of our skull. For instance, when we crunch a biscuit most of the sound is transmitted by vibration of the skull directly to the inner ear. This fact is used in the diagnosis of hearing loss; for instance, if someone can hear sounds more clearly when transmitted through the bone than through the ear-drum, then the problem lies in the middle ear. Violinists with middle ear disease may still be able to play, simply through transmission of sound through the skull from the instrument. Bone conduction hearing is important for normal speech since the voice is partly monitored through vibrations heard directly by the inner ear via the skull. Humming, for example, is largely heard through the bone of the skull. If airborne sounds are blotted out by placing fingers in the ears, the hum appears to get louder. Normally a speaker hears both air- and bone-conducted sounds. The listener, of course, hears only the air-conducted sounds; this explains why, when one hears a recording of one's own voice, it does not seem at all as one imagines it. The low frequency vibrations of our vocal cords are conducted to our own ears through the skull, making our voice sound much more powerful and impressive to ourselves. Consequently, a recording of our own voice often sounds rather thin and disappointing. The control of speaking and singing involves a complicated feedback system which allows us to continually adjust and correct the voice as we speak or sing and is intimately linked with changing the tension of our vocal cords if the pitch is wrong.

Much of the discussion in later chapters on the various conditions which give rise to hearing loss are connected with disturbances of the normal structure of the ear, and frequent reference will be made back to this chapter in the hope of making the disease processes more easily understood.

3

HEARING TESTS

The testing of infants and small children for deafness will be discussed in Chapter 7, while this chapter will deal with all the common hearing tests that might be carried out in an ear, nose, and throat (ENT) department. In practice, many people will have carried out their own basic hearing tests before coming to the department; for instance, they may have compared the sound of a ticking watch in the left and right ear, or their own hearing of various sounds with that of their friends or relatives. Although many family doctors carry out hearing tests, it is likely that referral to a specialist hospital department will be necessary.

VOICE TESTS

The tester will probably examine each ear individually and then both together by measuring roughly at what distance the patient can hear a whispered voice, a quiet conversational voice, and a loud conversational voice. It is important that the tester's face cannot be seen, to avoid the possibility of the patient lip-reading. The results might be recorded as follows:

left ear	whispered voice	0.6 m
right ear	quiet conversational voice	0.6 m

This gives an indication that the right ear is less efficient than the left, but it does not quantify the hearing loss.

This test is however rather crude and cannot be considered to be accurate.

TUNING FORK TESTS

Most doctors do not bother with the voice tests, and start off the examination of hearing by using a tuning fork test. This does not quantify the degree of the patient's hearing; however, it is extremely valuable in establishing whether the hearing loss originates from the middle or the inner ear. The usual tuning fork employed has a frequency of 512 Hz, which is at the lower end of the normal speech range. The doctor strikes the tuning fork, usually on his knee or elbow, to set it vibrating and then holds it first opposite the ear canal and then, with the base of the tuning fork applied to the bone immediately behind the ear (Plate II). The patient is then asked which of the two sounds he or she has heard as the loudest. In normal hearing the sound travelling down the ear-canal to the ear-drum, is heard better.

If, however, there is a malfunction of the *middle ear* (such as a hole in the ear-drum, fluid in the middle ear, or disruption or fixation of one of the ossicles), then the tuning fork appears loudest when placed on the bone behind the ear. From here the sound is transmitted via the skull directly to the inner ear.

With *inner ear* deafness on the other hand, the patient still hears the tuning fork better when sound is transmitted via the ear-canal and ear-drum. Provided the examiner's hearing is normal, a further simple test may then be done, in which the patient is asked to indicate when he can no longer hear the vibrating tuning fork. At this point the fork is quickly held up to the examiner's ear. If the examiner can still hear the sound then the patient's hearing is worse than the examiner's and the likely cause is an inner ear deafness.

A further test is for the vibrating tuning fork to be placed on the head at the centre of the forehead; the patient is asked in which ear the sound is heard the loudest (Plate III). If the right ear has an inner ear deafness, then because the left inner ear is the best hearing ear the sound will appear to be transmitted towards this side so the patient will say he can hear best on the left. If, on the other hand, the right ear has a middle ear deafness he will hear the tuning fork more loudly on the right side. This is because environmental 'background noise' in the room is 'filtered out' as it is not transmitted so easily through the ear-canal of the abnormal middle ear on this side. This lack of background 'masking' gives the impression that the patient can hear better through bone on the abnormal side.

These tests are very simple to perform and are extremely useful as a quick, reliable, and cheap test of hearing in adults and children over the age of 5 years. However, they do not give an absolute level of the patient's hearing but are rather an aid to diagnosing which part of the ear is faulty.

PURE-TONE AUDIOMETRY

The word 'audiometry' comes from the Latin *'audire'* meaning 'to hear' and the Greek word *'metrios'* meaning 'to measure'. An audiometer is a machine that can generate sound at an accurate level of loudness, measured as decibels (dB), and tone at specific frequencies (Hz or CPS). This sound can be altered in regular steps across the normal frequencies heard by the ear to produce a graphical represent-ation of the patient's hearing, which is called an 'audio-gram'.

In a hospital department the patient is placed in a room or booth which has been specially treated to exclude back-ground noise. The patient wears a pair of head-phones connecting him to the audiometer. A typical audiogram chart is shown in Fig. 4. Along the bottom are the usual frequencies used for the test (in Hz) and down the side is the loudness (in dB). The ears are tested separately and for each frequency the intensity of the sound delivered is altered in small steps until the patient indicates the quietest sound that he can hear. This is called the 'threshold of hearing' for that

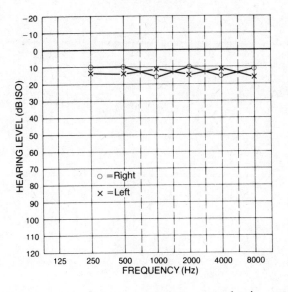

Fig. 4 Pure-tone audiogram showing normal air conduction hearing.

particular frequency and is recorded on the chart, usually using a circle for the right ear and a cross for the left. Wearing head-phones, of course, means the intensity is measured via the ear-canal as air-conducted sound. Just as with the tuning fork, bone conduction can also be measured, and for this the patient wears a small transmitter which is held in place by a head-band so that it is tightly applied to the bone behind the ear. The test is carried out in exactly the same way as described for the air conduction test and the result plotted using different symbols (Fig. 5).

If the tuning fork tests suggest that the patient can hear better when the sound is applied via the bone at the back of the ear, which would suggest middle ear deafness, the bone trace should be better than the air trace on the audiogram (Fig. 6). So instead of knowing only that the patient has a middle ear deafness, the doctor can discover the exact degree of deafness from the audiogram.

Nevertheless, various difficulties can occur during these

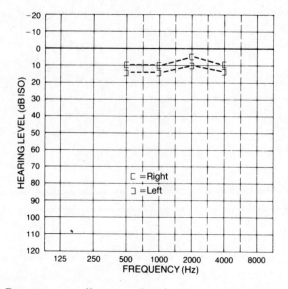

Fig. 5 Pure-tone audiogram showing normal bone (inner ear) hearing carried out using a sound source held on the bone behind the ear.

tests. For example, in very deaf people sound may be transmitted across the skull and may confuse the results of each ear being tested separately. To overcome this, a technique of 'masking' is used whereby a hissing noise is applied to the ear not being tested; this prevents cross-referral of sound.

Although pure-tone audiometry is helpful, none of us hears pure tones in real life. In this respect the test is artificial and so speech audiometry is sometimes used instead. This is slightly more complicated, but is particularly useful for demonstrating the patient's ability to hear the spoken word. A list of different words is transmitted through headphones from a tape recorder at known sound intensity; each word is simply repeated by the patient as it is heard. The percentage of correct answers is calculated and plotted on a chart. Provided that the sounds applied are loud enough, the patient can usually achieve nearly 100 per cent accurate scores in middle ear deafness; however, with inner ear deaf-

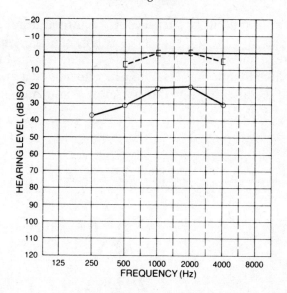

Fig. 6 Pure-tone audiogram of right middle ear deafness: the bone conduction is normal but the air (middle ear) conduction is reduced by 20dB.

ness, no matter how loud the intensity, the percentage score is never 100 per cent.

So far, the tests mentioned have been dependent on the patient's ability to say 'yes, I can hear it' or 'no, I cannot'. In the following sections, two tests are described which are automatic and do not require the co-operation of the patient.

TYMPANOMETRY

Tympanometry is particularly useful in children for diagnosing whether fluid is present in the middle ear; it relies on the elasticity of the ear-drum being measured. A tympanometer transmits a low frequency sound to the ear-drum and measures how much of it is reflected with a microphone. By changing the pressure in the ear-canal, the ear-drum can either be pushed in or sucked out. A normal drum is least stiff when it is in the middle position, that is, when the pressure on either side of the drum is equal. A tympanogram pattern like that in Fig. 7 is obtained, showing that at atmospheric pressure the ear-drum is most compliant (floppy).

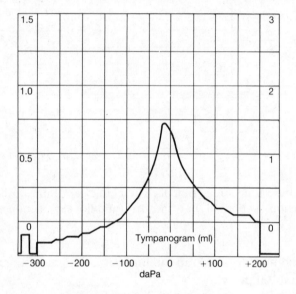

Fig. 7 Normal tympanogram: the maximum movement of the eardrum occurs at atmospheric pressure, hence the peak at 0 on the lower scale.

However, the middle ear is full of fluid then, no matter what the pressure change in the ear canal, the ear-drum will not move. The amount of reflected sound does not change so a flat line is obtained on the tympanogram (Fig. 8). This information is invaluable in the diagnosis of 'glue ear' (Chapter 9). To carry out this test, it is necessary to have an airtight seal in the ear-canal so that the pressure can be altered accurately. Plates IVa and b show children having such a test, in which the tympanometer is connected to an auroscope with a special sealed ear-canal insert.

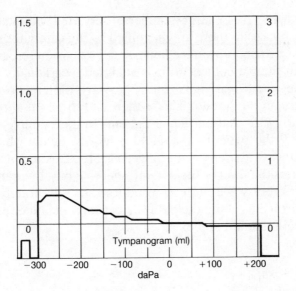

Fig. 8 Tympanogram of 'glue ear': a flat line occurs due to the ear being full of fluid (glue), preventing ear-drum movement no matter what the pressure is.

ELECTRIC RESPONSE AUDIOMETRY

In practice this test is used only in rare circumstances, compared with the huge number of people requiring hearing tests. It may, however, be extremely useful in children with multihandicap who are unable to undergo pure-tone audiometry, or in the diagnosis of some of the rarer diseases that affect the inner ear. The electric response audiometer is able to pick up minute electrical impulses generated by the inner ear, auditory nerve, and parts of the brain when sound is applied to that ear. The problem is that there is an enormous amount of other electrical activity in the brain occurring all the time; the most important part of the machine is therefore a computer that can average out all the background electrical activity of the brain and magnify the tiny responses produced by the inner ear and auditory nerve.

The ear receives a large number of repeated sound stimuli; the responses to these are magnified by the computer so that a wave pattern is produced on a small television screen. The level of the patient's hearing is analysed by gradually reducing the sound test signal until the wave pattern no longer appears on the screen. This is then said to be the threshold of hearing for that particular patient. In the example shown in Fig. 9 the patient's threshold is 60 dB, below which the typical wave pattern is no longer visible. This test not only measures the level of the patient's hearing but, by examining the different wave patterns produced, can accurately diagnose problems along the pathway between the inner ear and the brain, should any exist.

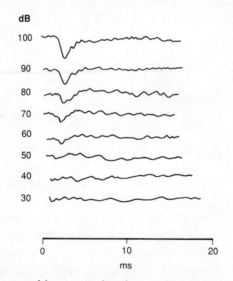

Fig. 9 Electrocochleogram showing typical wave form petering out at 60 dB—the minimum level heard by the subject.

This test requires no co-operation from the patient and is sometimes used when ordinary tests of hearing are not conclusive, for example in babies, mental or physical handicap, or for diagnosis of rare inner ear, nerve, or brain problems associated with deafness.

4

TYPES OF DEAFNESS

Just as the ear is divided structurally into different parts, so afflictions of these various parts cause quite different types of hearing loss. It is essential to distinguish between these types as the treatment is totally different.

If obstruction to hearing is a result of some abnormality in the outer and/or middle ears, the deafness is said to be of a *conductive* type. If the inner ear is affected a *sensory* deafness results, and if the nerve of hearing is involved then a *neural* hearing loss occurs. More usually these two latter groups are lumped together under the term *sensorineural* because it requires very sophisticated hearing tests to distinguish between them. The essential distinction made is therefore between a conductive and a sensorineural hearing loss.

From all practical points of view it is often possible to treat and hopefully cure, either medically or surgically, a conductive hearing loss, which most commonly results from problems in the middle ear. Sensorineural hearing loss, on the other hand, sadly cannot be cured but only helped by a hearing aid (see Chapter 18), although exceptions occur in some people with Menière's disease (Chapter 13) and some cases of sudden deafness (Chapter 14). There are also some important causes of sensorineural deafness which, although very rare, if not diagnosed and treated may lead to more debilitating problems; for example in the case of a completely benign tumour (acoustic neuroma) that occasionally arises on the auditory nerve.

CHARACTERISTICS OF CONDUCTIVE DEAFNESS

Hearing tests on people with conductive deafness show the inner ear or nerve function to be normal but the air conduction to be reduced (Fig. 6), and medical or surgical treatment, or just amplification (raising the voice or issuing a temporary hearing aid), gives excellent speech understanding and restores hearing levels to normal. The voice of a person with a conductive deafness is usually quiet. This is because sound generated by one's own voice appears louder owing to direct conduction through the skull into the inner ear—just as the tuning fork tests described in the last chapter show that in middle ear deafness a tuning fork held on the skull appears louder than one held at the ear canal. Because of the apparent increase in volume of the voice, it tends to be used more quietly since the sufferer thinks he is shouting. Some types of middle ear deafness (notably otosclerosis) exhibit another peculiar feature in that there is an apparent ability to hear better in noisy surroundings. This was first described in the seventeenth century by Dr Thomas Willis who told the story of a woman whose hearing was improved if a drum was beaten regularly while she was in conversation, and records how her husband kept a drummer just so that he could have a reasonable conversation with her! The simple explanation for this phenomenon is that in noisy surroundings the speaker tends to raise the voice and in this way overcomes conductive hearing loss.

CHARACTERISTICS OF SENSORINEURAL DEAFNESS

Sensorineural deafness on the other hand is very often accompanied by different degrees of inner ear or nerve function failure for specific frequencies, most usually worse in the high frequencies (Fig. 10), which are associated with consonants of speech such as 'T', 'D', 'S', etc. Vowels are low frequency sounds heard in the low frequency end of the hearing range. If hearing for consonants is reduced, speech discrimination is poor; simply amplifying the sound by raising the voice or using a non-selective hearing aid in fact overamplifies the often normal low frequencies in an effort to improve the high frequency loss and results in a noisy jumble. Another characteristic of sensorineural deafness is that it is quite commonly accompanied by a phenomenon called 'recruitment', whereby sound becomes distorted and occasionally painful when the voice is raised, giving rise to the familiar comment 'don't shout at me, I'm not deaf!' The voice in sensorineural deafness is unlike that in conductive deafness in that it is frequently raised—we are all familiar with the elderly man who appears to be shouting when we are using a normal conversational voice. This is because he cannot monitor the volume of his own voice as sound is not

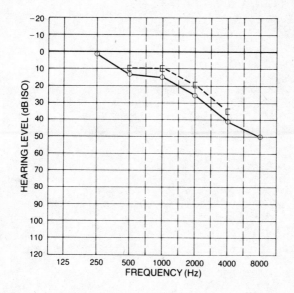

Fig. 10 Pure-tone audiometry: typical high frequency hearing loss in right ear.

fed back into his inner ears owing to hearing loss in them.

The above is a simplified account of the differences between conductive and sensorineural deafness; the following chapters go into these conditions in greater detail and explain how they may be managed.

Part I

CHILDHOOD PROBLEMS

5

THE DEVELOPMENT OF NORMAL
HEARING, SPEECH, AND LANGUAGE

Variations in normal hearing responses and deviations of speech and language development may be the first clues that a child suffers from hearing loss. The most vital need in the management of the deaf child is early diagnosis, which unfortunately does not often happen at present. The brain goes through a series of developmental stages at each of which it is best at learning certain things; for instance a young child can hold and play with a cricket bat or tennis racquet with the left or right hand, a task which is usually awkward for an adult; left and right handedness on the piano are also easier for a child to overcome than for an adult learning for the first time. The brain is 'plastic' at a young age and easily moulded to acquire different skills. Listening for the purpose of learning to speak is an early part of brain development and, if a hearing-impaired child is identified early, then correct stimulus at that stage gives him a much greater chance of reasonable speech development than if diagnosis is delayed. A child diagnosed before 6 months of age has a huge advantage over one in whom diagnosis is delayed until 18 months.

Table 1 is presented as a check-list for parents; if their child deviates from the norm then professional advice should be sought. There is a wide variation in what is considered 'normal' and most cases of deviation are accounted for by this variation. No professional minds checking a child's hearing for normality, but failing to test a deaf child until it is too late to help is a tragedy. Whether health care professionals like it or not, parents are the most accurate indicators of whether their child has a hearing problem and it is a foolish doctor or health visitor who ignores a parent who says 'I am worried about my baby's hearing'.

Age	Response to sound	Speech and language
0–4 months	Reflex startle. 'Stills' and listens (stilling = stopping gurgling, crying, or wriggling in response to sound)	Different sounds for hunger, comfort, and pain
By 4 months	'Stills' and smiles to parents voices	Vocalizes in response to louder sounds only
By 6 months	Turns head to source sound inconsistently. Responds to lower volume sound	Gurgles with pleasure
By 9 months	Turns accurately to locate sound source at head level. May not look up or down to find sounds above or below head level	Tuneful babble (da da, ma ma, etc.) Occasionally copies sounds
By 12 months	Localizes sound on any plane. Understands 'No' and a few objects	May attempt to say or repeat one or two words
By 18 months	Responds to questions, e.g. where are your shoes?, when he will point to his feet	Says 12 or so single words, usually children's names, 'cat', 'dog', 'car', etc.
By 24 months	Picks out correct toys when asked. Answers simple questions	Joining of two words in meaningful way. Intonation and rhythm to speech
By 36 months	Turns to sound only if interested	Well-formed sentences

This table is intended only as a rough guide and it should be emphasized that there is often considerable variation in what is considered normal. The most remarkable feature is the consistency with which hearing and language development occurs. The new-born child has an inbuilt ability to react and to have 'contact' with his parents from birth. This innate ability is a feature only of the human race and the early stages of language (under 6 months), which include 'cooing', gurgling, and crying, do not seem to be dependent on normal hearing. Even severely deaf babies will make these early attempts at language.

The development of language is dependent on the ability to understand, to think, and to express thoughts as speech. Understanding and thinking are very much interlinked and together build up an internal memory of concepts that can be drawn upon and expressed as speech. It is quite normal for a child to understand a good deal more than he is capable of expressing. Speech delay is a common reason for referral for specialist help. Very often it is found that the child understands everything that is said and obviously has no hearing loss but for some reason is not stimulated enough to reproduce his thoughts as speech. It may be that if a 2-year-old child can ask for a glass of milk by pointing and saying 'ugh' and the milk is given him, he may think 'well what's the point of talking if all I have to do is to point and grunt!' Boys are frequently far behind girls in their speech development at this stage.

So far we have considered only normal variations. Abnormal factors can also influence speech and language development considerably, the most obvious being hearing loss. The more severe the deafness, the greater is the effect on language development; but even mild degrees of conductive deafness (for instance glue ear—see Chapter 9) are thought in some cases to have a significant effect. With a hearing-impaired child, intonation may remain flat with less rhythm and variation, and sounds such as 'ma ma' and 'da da' which are used from 8–9 months are eagerly interpreted as meaningful 'words' by parents. Just as the younger deaf child will coo etc. the older child may continue to use such 'words' indiscriminately for some time.

Sight is the other main sense to affect language. If an object cannot be seen, then it is difficult to associate it with its name; thus children with sight problems are not infrequently language delayed.

Intelligence obviously comes into the ability of a child to acquire language. A low innate IQ score or specific brain damage will result in retardation of language.

The child's environment is another particularly important factor. A deprived child lacking in stimulation, whether it be a lack of parental contact or lack of experience, will have delayed language acquisition. The detrimental effect of withdrawing 'mother–child bonding', such as might occur in a severely ill baby hospitalized for the first few months of its life, has not been fully proved, but care needs to be taken by hospital personnel to stimulate their little charges and ensure that as much natural development as possible takes place.

We must all strive to identify the child with hearing loss much earlier; if this chapter and the check-list go some way in helping to achieve this, then its purpose will have been worthwhile.

6

CAUSES OF CHILDHOOD DEAFNESS

The causes of deafness can be split into conductive and sensorineural types (see Chapter 4). Conductive losses, from whatever cause, are far less serious than sensorineural ones since the inner ear and auditory nerve are normal and by some means (i.e. surgery or hearing aids) near-normal speech can be made to reach the brain for interpretation. Thus, in a child born with a conductive deafness, speech usually develops normally. In those born with sensorineural deafness or who develop it prior to speech development there are serious implications for the development of speech. However, even in profound sensorineural deafness, hearing aids and effective teaching make speech development possible if early detection occurs. The key, however, is early detection; the following chapters will emphasize this point.

CLASSIFICATION

It is usual to divide the causes of deafness into those that are inherited through the genes, such as might occur if two deaf people were to marry and have children, and those that are acquired during pregnancy, from such causes as infections like rubella (German measles), certain hearing-damaging drugs, and birth trauma. Other illnesses, such as meningitis in the prespeech stage of life (i.e. under 9 months) can have a profound effect on hearing. The commonest cause of childhood hearing loss by far is 'glue ear' and this is discussed in a separate chapter (Chapter 9). This is a conductive hearing loss, nearly always occurring after speech has developed; provided it is recognized and managed correctly then speech, language, and educational attainment should not be affected. Other conductive causes of hearing loss that occur later in childhood, such as a perforated ear-drum or disruption of the ossicular chain (malleus, incus, and stapes), are also considered in a later chapter (Chapter 11).

Conductive deafness will not be mentioned further in this chapter, which will concentrate on sensorineural deafness. This occurs in about one in a thousand live births and the severity is very variable. However, thanks to better antenatal and neonatal care of small babies and vaccination for rubella, the number of cases being reported is dropping. There are now fewer pupils in schools for the hard of hearing.

CAUSES OF SENSORINEURAL DEAFNESS

Unknown

Of all reported causes of deafness in childhood, the biggest single group is 'cause unknown'. These cases are always sensorineural and comprise at least 25–30 per cent of all cases. They are labelled 'unknown' because despite every effort to sort out the possible causes, which would include a careful history of any family deafness, problems in early pregnancy, and detailed investigation of the child's early life, including possible causative factors at birth, no reasonable cause can be found. This group will therefore probably remain with us as a hard core of new cases each year and there is little that can be done to reduce the incidence. The problem with this group is that there is nothing that might predict a hearing loss, whereas there are many other factors that are known to cause deafness and if detected either before or at birth result in the child being put on an 'at risk' register. This register alerts all health workers to check doubly that the child is developing normally and should ensure that any hearing loss is detected quickly. This is not possible with the unknown group; they are therefore likely to present a little later, with detrimental results for speech development. It may well be that these hearing losses are genetically determined but only inheritance of the deafness by the next generation will confirm this.

Genetic causes

The ear is fully formed by the time that the fetus is 3 months old and genetic influences may completely stop development of the ear or cause maldevelopment in its structure. Intermarriage between people who have an unknown cause of sensorineural deafness may produce deaf offspring. Another group that is causing increasing concern is that of related intermarriage in certain races. There are also a whole host of very rare syndromes with complicated names which cause various abnormalities of the outer, middle, or inner ear. The outer and middle ears are formed from a totally different part of the developing fetus to the inner ear, which is part of the nervous system; yet genetic influences can damage not only inner ear function, but also the construction of the outer and middle ear. If the inner ear is damaged a severe sensorineural hearing loss will result. It is possible, however, to develop perfectly normal inner ears with grossly abnormal external and middle ears, resulting in a conductive deafness, which is much more treatable. There is, of course, no difficulty in recognizing children born with grossly abnormal external ears. With sophisticated hearing tests and/or X-rays, including computer scanning, it is also possible to determine whether or not the structure and function of the middle and inner ears are normal. If both ears are affected these investigations should be carried out early to determine whether the child is likely to have a major problem in speech acquisition, and whether anything can be done about it, so that the parents can be counselled as soon as possible.

Genetic causes can also show their effect after birth. In one particular type, often called *hereditary cochlear degeneration*, children may be born with normal hearing but later in childhood the cochlea (inner ear) begins to undergo gradual degeneration. Many of these children will develop speech while their hearing is still normal but by the time they reach early teenage life they have a severe deafness. Unfortunately, there is at present no treatment to prevent this happening. Another cause of late onset sensorineural deafness is associated with a rare kidney disease (*Alport's syndrome*). Again this results in progressive deterioration of the sensorineural hearing, usually in the high frequencies and, although it occurs in families, different members of that family often have different degrees of hearing loss.

Acquired causes

Before birth

As discussed above, the first 3 months of pregnancy are critical to the development of the ear and the influence of certain infections and drugs are particularly important.

Infections. The classic infection causing deafness is of course rubella. In the 1950s this infection was responsible for about 20 per cent of severely hearing-impaired children. Recently, however, community screening of teenage girls has been employed to identify those who have not caught rubella naturally, and therefore not developed immunity to it. Vaccination of those not immune has caused the incidence to drop rapidly. This is one of the true success stories of modern preventative medicine and has had the effect of reducing the numbers of deaf children requiring special education. The vaccination programme of course varies from area to area around the world but, theoretically, rubella deafness could be eradicated with 100 per cent screening and appropriate immunization. However, this will probably never be completely possible. Rubella deafness may also be associated with other defects which make up the full rubella syndrome; these include heart abnormalities, blindness, and a degree of mental retardation. If a mother develops rubella during the first 3 months of pregnancy the probability is high that the child will suffer some degree of sensorineural deafness; then difficult moral and ethical problems with regard to termination of pregnancy occasionally arise. The deafness in rubella is very variable but it is always sensorineural. There are also cases of children born excreting the rubella virus in their urine who have apparently normal hearing at 9 months, but who by the age of 2 years are profoundly deaf. It is therefore very important that, if rubella is suspected in early pregnancy, blood is taken from the baby to test antibody levels to the virus so that a very careful follow-up can be arranged for the child.

Another virus that has been implicated is the Cytomegalovirus. This causes a very mild, flu-like illness; it sometimes occurs in early pregnancy and may be a cause of deafness in the new-born child. This is of considerably rarer occurrence than rubella and, considering it is a very common virus to which most normal people have antibodies and are therefore protected, it probably does not require further consideration.

Drugs.   The classic drug that caused severe hearing problems was Thalidomide®. This was a drug that had been given for morning sickness in the first three months of pregnancy until it was seen to cause disastrous defects in some babies. The most obvious abnormalities were defects in upper and lower limb development, but a large proportion of babies also had severe outer, middle, and occasionally inner ear defects. All drugs should be used with precaution in the first three months of pregnancy and there is good evidence that certain antibiotics are risky, particularly those in the aminoglycoside group of which Streptomycin is the parent drug.

X-rays.   Radiotherapy being given for therapeutic reasons to women not known to be pregnant has produced abnormalities in the fetus, including deafness. It is therefore very unwise to carry out unnecessary X-rays in the first three months of confirmed or suspected pregnancy and special precautions should be taken to avoid any form of radiation to the abdomen.

Thyroid disease.   It is difficult to know whether some forms of cretinism are due to maternal thyroid disease from iodine deficiency or whether they are genetically determined. However, special interest should be paid to the child born to the mother with thyroid disease because early treatment to replace deficient thyroid hormone can prevent all the stigma of cretinism, including deafness.

Hearing loss acquired at birth

All new-born babies have a mild conductive deafness due to fluid in their middle ears. However, this clears very quickly and is of no importance. It is simply caused by the presence of the amniotic fluid in which the baby has been living in the uterus for the past 9 months. Sensorineural hearing loss is, however, associated with problems at birth, particularly prematurity. A full-term baby is delivered after 40 weeks in the mother's uterus, but it is now possible, thanks to special baby units and medical expertise, to keep 26-week-old premature babies alive. However, prematurity has its own special hazards, particularly immature lungs, and this may well lead to lack of oxygen transfer with lowering of the normal oxygen levels in the blood. The inner ear is particularly sensitive to lack of oxygen and it is normally the cells in the inner ear associated with high frequency hearing that are affected. However, despite the large number of premature babies that are now being looked after, many of whom have spells where they are short of oxygen, the incidence of deafness in good neonatal units is surprisingly low.

Jaundice in the new-born baby is much rarer than it used

to be thanks to development in the prevention of Rhesus incompatibility. In addition to the ABO blood groups there is another subdivision into Rhesus positive and Rhesus negative type. A Rhesus negative mother may carry a Rhesus positive fetus. There is mixing of the bloods across the placenta at birth and the mother will then produce antibodies to the Rhesus positive blood received from the child. The first child is not affected by this but the antibodies remain in the mother's blood and if a second child is born its blood may be damaged by these; the result of which is jaundice. If the jaundice becomes severe it puts the hearing very much at risk, and a high frequency sensorineural deafness can occur. However, this problem can now be overcome. The mother is given anti-D gammaglobulin after her first delivery which effectively prevents antibody formation against Rhesus positive blood. In the past the only treatment was to exchange the baby's blood completely to remove maternal antibodies and this often had to be done on two or three occasions, presenting a very serious problem. It is now a rarity, as is the deafness associated with this type of jaundice.

Antibiotics may have to be given to severely sick, premature babies; unfortunately, the most effective of the antibiotics are also likely to be those which can cause ear damage. Clinicians are well aware of the risk and the blood levels of these antibiotics are carefully monitored to make sure they do not exceed a toxic level. Nevertheless, occasional cases are reported of hearing damage from antibiotics given in neonatal units.

Other causes that have been implicated at birth have included noise from the machinery working the incubators and ventilators in the neonatal units. However, the evidence for this is not strong and, as has been mentioned before, despite the large number of children passing through these units, only a tiny minority are deafened.

Hearing loss occurring during infancy

It is essential to have good hearing for the acquisition of

speech, the development of which was described in Chapter 5. In most children the first word of speech is produced between the ages of nine months and one year.

The major problem is once again sensorineural hearing loss and the most important cause is meningitis. Meningitis may cause deafness in a number of different ways, including direct infection of the inner ear; occasionally deafness is secondary to the need for antibiotics to treat certain forms of meningitis. Certainly, all children who have had meningitis must have their hearing checked when the disease is cured.

Measles and mumps can also cause hearing loss. Mumps is peculiar in that it usually causes total deafness in one ear only.

SUMMARY

Although there will always be a hard core of about 30 per cent of cases in which no cause is known for hearing loss in childhood, the overall incidence is dropping. This is because of better community care in the prevention of rubella, increased expertise by those running special care baby units, and the conquering of Rhesus incompatibility problems. However, hearing loss in childhood will never be eradicated completely and the key to successful management is early identification (see Chapter 7).

7

ASSESSMENT OF THE YOUNG CHILD'S HEARING

As discussed in the last chapter, the reason for assessing children's hearing is to detect those with impairment as early in life as possible since hearing is vital for the normal acquisition of speech and language.

Unfortunately, our success at early detection is decidedly inadequate. A recent European Economic Community (EEC) survey suggested that only 25 per cent of hearing-impaired children were identified before 12 months and 45 per cent were still undiagnosed by three years of age. This is clearly grossly unsatisfactory. Many people feel that parental suspicion is the most accurate indication of early hearing loss. Part of the failure of screening for deafness may be due either to ineffectual testing or to too many children slipping through the screening net. It is therefore essential to improve baby-screening services for the identification of the hearing-impaired child.

There are two forms of childhood hearing tests—screening and diagnostic. All children should have screening tests and if they fall below the norm they should then have diagnostic tests to establish the type and exact extent of their hearing loss.

SCREENING TESTS

The ideal screen would be to have every new-born child monitored by an automatic electric response audiometer (see below) shortly after birth or before leaving hospital.

This would give a print-out of his or her hearing abilities. The test would have to be as simple and quick to perform as a routine electrocardiogram (ECG) and could be part of the standard paediatric examination already carried out on all children. As yet, no such machine exists, although various devices including the *crib-o-gram* and *auditory response cradle* are getting near. However, they are still too time consuming for routine use. These machines work by measuring changes in heart and respiration rate and body movements in response to sound stimulation.

At present most screening has to rely on observable reaction to sound rather than an automatic response generated as above. The exception would be the at-risk children. In these the time spent doing electric response audiometry soon after birth is well worth while because of the potential number of hearing-impaired children it might yield. At-risk children would include those with a family history of sensorineural deafness, those whose mothers may have had contact with rubella in early pregnancy, and those who had particularly difficult birth problems or a stormy beginning to their lives, which may have included prolonged hospitalization in a special baby care unit.

In most children, screening takes place between six and eight months of age and relies on the ability of the child to turn to the source of sound. This type of screening is called *distraction testing*.

Distraction tests

These tests need to be carried out in comfortable, soundproofed rooms without too much in the room to overinterest the child. They rely very heavily on a relaxed child, an acute observer, and a cunning tester—this immediately gives three sources of error! The arrangement is shown in Fig. 11.

The observer first attracts the child's interest with an object such as a toy; then the tester introduces a sound source behind and to either side of the child. The child's

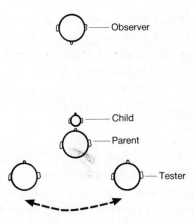

Fig. 11 Positioning of parent with child, tester, and observer.

response may be an obvious turning of the head. However, in younger infants a blink, cessation of cooing, or change in expression may be all there is to indicate a response. This type of testing requires a great deal of competence and is one which is very difficult for the large numbers of those who are responsible for screening to acquire skilfully. The sounds used for the test seem rather primitive but it has to be remembered that babies do not like boring pure tones as generated by an audiometer (Chapter 3); the source has to be interesting to the child as well as being of known frequency and loudness to the tester. It is important to test for low, middle, and high frequency hearing. Low frequency (500 Hz) can be tested using the sound 'oooo', mid frequency (1 kHz) with humming 'mmmm', and high frequency (3 kHz) by 'ssss'. Rattles are readily available for high frequency testing (the Manchester rattle). Frequency-specific chime bars can be used and more recently 'warble tone' devices have been available. The volume of sound being presented at a known distance from the child comes with experience and by checking it with a loudness meter (decibel meter). These may not sound very scientific tests but, carried out well and in conjunction with the parent's opinion, they are excellent screening tests and can be carried out in 'well baby clinics'. A failed test should lead to a repeat test two or three weeks later; if this too is failed then the child should be referred, if necessary, for more specific diagnostic tests.

Co-operation testing

Co-operation testing is appropriate, and indeed necessary, for screening older children since at 12–30 months children develop the ability to ignore some sound stimuli deliberately and tend to gaze around the room rather than localizing sound. To maintain interest, testing is done as a game. Usually the child is encouraged to respond to simple instructions, for instance putting a brick in a box or a ring on a peg. This holds his interest and, while the game is going on, a sound source is introduced behind and to the side of the child. In his relaxed state, the child will often respond by localizing the test sound. As the child reaches 30 months, this type of testing can be changed so that when a sound source is presented he will respond by putting a brick in a box or a ring on a peg. By varying the volume of sound and its frequency a rudimentary audiogram can be built up. This is known as *conditioning audiometry*.

Electric screening tests

Mention was made earlier of electrophysiological tests that were too complex for routine widespread screening use. However, a response known as the *postauricular muscle response* is currently being assessed as a useful screening device. So far, assessment with this instrument suggests that it is quick and easy to perform by personnel with limited training. It relies on the fact, that just as dogs prick up their ears when they hear sound, so muscles behind the ear in the human will give minute twitches in response to sound. These can be recorded by this machine. This quick screening test indicates either a pass or a fail, and if the child passes it it is assumed he has enough hearing to develop normal speech and language. The advantage of this test, if it does become widely available, is that it does not require particularly quiet conditions or a still child.

DIAGNOSTIC TESTS

A child who fails screening will be referred for diagnostic tests, usually in a fully equipped ear, nose, and throat (ENT) department. It is usual, first, to repeat the screening tests. If these are failed again then diagnostic tests appropriate to the child's age will be carried out. The commonest cause of deafness is glue ear (Chapter 9) and an ENT doctor will always need to examine the ear.

Tympanometry (Chapter 3) can be carried out and does not require the co-operation of the young child. This will give a characteristic shape and trace if middle ear fluid is present. However, if it is normal, audiometry is the next stage since the hearing loss is most likely to be sensorineural (Chapter 4) and it is necessary to know the degree of deafness across all frequencies. If the child is aged three years or over then conditioning audiometry will be required; this is usually done free field (Plate V). This is followed by puretone audiometry (Chapter 3) where the child wears earphones in a sound-proofed booth (Plate VI).

Speech tests

These tests are important not so much for assessing the level of hearing but to discover whether the child's understanding of speech is up to scratch. Most babies of 18 months or older will point, if asked, in response to questions such as 'where's mummy's nose or eyes?', etc. The voice level of the tester can be measured and the mouth covered to prevent lip reading. Tests may become more sophisticated and appropriate to language development and may include picture tests where the child indicates one object from a set of similar-sounding ones (Plate VII).

Once a child reaches the age of five or so, the tests are the same as for adults (see Chapter 3).

Electric response audiometry

Electric response audiometry (ERA) has been one of the major advances in audiology in the last 20 years. It enables the tester to monitor electrical responses to sound from the cochlea, auditory nerve, or brain without the co-operation of the child. Thus it is useful in multi-handicap, mental retardation, or in uncertain cases below the age where routine audiometry is possible. It is time consuming and, as mentioned above, is not yet available, except possibly as the postauricular muscle response, as a routine screening test.

Postauricular muscle response

This has already been mentioned earlier and, although it may be useful as a screening test, it is not accurate enough to be a diagnostic one.

Electrocochleography

This test is carried out by recording activity from the cochlea. A needle electrode is passed through the ear-drum so that it rests on the outside of the cochlea. It is obvious from this description that, in a child, a general anaesthetic is necessary, which is a disadvantage. However, it can give both accurate results and the opportunity to assess the middle ear and treat glue ear at the same time, if this is also present.

Brain stem audiometry

This test uses the same equipment as electrocochleography but electrodes are placed at strategic places on the skull to pick up reflexes passing from the auditory nerve into the brain. This requires the child to be very still and quiet and can mean sedation or general anaesthetia, which is a disadvantage.

There is no reason to carry out electrical tests unless conventional testing as described earlier is not possible or its validity is questioned.

Other assessment methods

It is always a good rule when a child is born with one defect to assume there may be others. As will be discussed in Chapter 8, one of the more efficient ways of managing children with sensorineural hearing loss is to use the multidisciplinary approach in which many specialists are involved who will initially be checking for other defects. These specialists will include eye doctors, neurologists, children's doctors, and genetic experts.

Blood tests may be useful for the diagnosis of rubella or certain other viruses, and thyroid hormone levels are sometimes routinely checked.

X-rays can be helpful, especially the newer forms of computer tomography (CT) because they accurately delineate the anatomy of the middle and inner ears. This may be of vital importance to future reconstructive surgery in those unfortunate babies born with malformed ears.

This chapter is intended to give a brief description of the methods used in assessing a child with hearing loss and the assessment is very much intertwined with management (discussed in the next chapter).

8

THE MANAGEMENT OF THE CHILD HANDICAPPED BY HEARING LOSS

THE PARENTS

Parents will usually be deeply shocked on finding out that their child has a sensorineural hearing loss and before the latter can be fitted with hearing aids they may need to be helped. Parents suffer from a variety of emotions which go through a series of stages: from shock and lack of acceptance, to anger, and then eventually to acceptance. They are all natural emotions and need to be handled by the health care professionals with understanding. The lack-of-acceptance stage often includes demands for second opinions and the professionals should not feel insulted. In most cases, further opinions only serve to confuse the parents and the sooner the stage of acceptance is reached, so that treatment of the child can be carried out, the better. Parents must be made to feel that they are not alone and local deaf child/parent groups such as the local branch of the National Deaf Children's Society can be very helpful in allaying fears. Counselling of parents is important and it does not matter much which of the many professionals who look after hearing-impaired children do this; however, consistent advice is essential.

Once the parents have accepted the hearing loss, most are only too keen to do all they can to help the development of the child's language—their first and main concern is often 'will my child be able to speak?' Many centres run a multi-disciplinary approach to the management and this may involve doctors specializing in children's ear, and eye diseases, as well as teachers of the deaf, speech therapists, psychologists, and hearing aid technicians. All these people are necessary to give an overall assessment of the child and to answer expertly the parents' many questions. Provided they reinforce each other's opinions, this arrangement is of great benefit and encouragement to the parents. Especially in the early stages, teaching is very much the role of the parents and a good relationship with the specialist teacher of the deaf, who will visit the home and advise, is essential. Very often long-lasting friendships develop between teacher and parent and this can only be an advantage for the child's educational development.

Advice must not appear to be conflicting; there are, however, differences of opinion as to which hearing aids, which type of school, and which type of communication is best. There are no hard-and-fast rules and confidence will be eroded if there is argument amongst the professionals!

THE CHILD

Hearing aids

As soon as possible after the diagnosis of sensorineural deafness, hearing aids need to be fitted. It does not matter if the severity of deafness has not yet been established, since in the early stages absolute accuracy is not possible; the important aim is to get sound to the child. Acceptance of the aids by the parents is often the key to the child's acceptance of them. Fortunately, total deafness is extremely rare. Nearly always hearing aid amplification will be helpful and the younger the child is when one is fitted the better is the eventual speech and language development. A full description of hearing aid fitting and different types of aids will be found in Chapter 18 and only an outline will be given here.

Range of hearing aids

There is an enormous range of hearing aids available; in the

UK, the National Health Service carries a wide variety of instruments to fit most needs. However, if a particular aid manufactured commercially is thought to be necessary to correct the child's hearing loss, this can be arranged. It is therefore important to leave the choice of model to the expert.

Because babies have very floppy ears, 'behind-the-ear' aids are too heavy and will keep falling out. It is therefore normal to begin with a 'body-worn' aid. Here the main components are in a box which is worn around the chest in a harness, and are connected by a wire to the small plastic moulded ear-pieces (*moulds*) worn inside the ears. The power output varies enormously between different aids (see Chapter 18); normally a fairly low-powered instrument will be chosen at first and changed if necessary as more information becomes available as to the degree of the child's hearing loss. In very rare instances when a child is born without external ears, bone-conducting hearing aids can be used. As children grow their ears become stiffer; in most instances, they will then be fitted with postaural (behind-the-ear) aids which are usually more cosmetically acceptable. Two hearing aids are probably better then one for localization purposes.

However, there are problems apart from the floppy ears already mentioned, especially '*feedback*'. This is a squealing sound emitted from the aid; it is often due to poorly fitting moulds allowing sound to feed back to the hearing aid microphone from the ear-canal. The more powerful the aid, the more liable this is to happen. By separating the microphone from the ear-mould, as in a 'body-worn' aid, this problem is overcome. So it may be necessary to keep 'body-worn' instruments if powerful hearing aids are necessary. Lack of squealing is reliant on well-made, well-fitting moulds and, since children are still growing, it is not surprising their ears enlarge and loosen these. The making of frequent new moulds is therefore the rule.

Radio aids

Radio aids have one huge advantage over conventional ones, especially in the classroom: the significant reduction in unwanted background noise. The teacher or parent wears a small radio microphone transmitter and the child a receiver. This may be either a slightly bulky, body-worn box or a connection directly to the child's 'behind-the-ear' aid. Only sound generated by the teacher will be received and this is not affected by the child's position in the class, which allows him free mobility.

Another teaching aid that reduces background sound is the so-called *group hearing aid*. Here each child in the class has headphones which are individually adjusted to his or her hearing loss. These are connected to a communal amplifier into which is fed the teacher's voice from a microphone. The only disadvantage with this system is the lack of mobility because of all the connecting wires!

EDUCATION

The hope with every deaf child is that eventually, through correct management, he will be able to communicate with and integrate fully into everyday society. This is not always possible and there are many reasons for this, the most obvious being the extent of the deafness. Other factors include the age of onset of the deafness, that is, whether speech had been learnt prior to the acquisition of the hearing loss, intelligence, the ability to use residual hearing, and the motivation of the child and especially the parents.

The subject of education of the deaf could fill several books, and already does, so this is intended merely as an outline of the services available. There are three systems of education used for the hearing-impaired child—mainstream (integration into 'normal' schools), partially hearing units (units for hearing-impaired children with specialist teachers

attached to the normal school), and schools for the deaf
(full-time residential schools for hearing-impaired children
run by specialist teachers of the deaf).

Preschool children

In most cases, education of the preschool child is carried out
at home and most areas run a peripatetic teaching and
counselling service. The object of this is to give realistic
information to support the parents, to help the child benefit
from amplification, to advise on the expectations, and to
maximize all aspects of normal development. Hearing aid
management, explaining the problem of background noise,
and establishing which parts of the child's hearing is deficient
with regard to speech development are all very important.
Regular support to the parents at this stage is also of vital
importance, as is the opportunity to mix with normal-hearing
children, and there may well be local playgroups or nursery
schools which are particularly suitable.

School age

Deaf children can be educated in a large variety of ways, but
there is a very definite and welcome move towards integration of hearing-impaired with normal-hearing children. This
of course depends on the degree of deafness and varies as
the child progresses through the educational system, integration increasing with age. Educational help ranges from
hearing aid provision and placement in ordinary classes to
special residential schools for the severely deafened. Partially
hearing units (PHU) in the UK fill the gap between these
extremes. These are buildings attached to a main school that
are specially adapted for the hearing impaired; they have a
specialized teacher of the deaf in charge. Children will spend
a variable amount of time in these units while they integrate
into mainstream schooling where possible. Once children
have graduated from the PHU and are fully integrated, then

extra help, sometimes outside school hours, is usually necessary from peripatetic teachers of the deaf. Teachers of mainstream classes may need to be taught to accept the wearing of radio microphones and be educated in the special needs of their deaf charges. Speech therapy lessons may also be required.

The object of the modern approach to educating the hearing-impaired child is to avoid social isolation and to improve communication so that eventually, whatever the degree of hearing loss, that child will be able to make his way in society. Good relations between teachers and parents are essential and both need to be adaptable to the changing needs of the hearing-impaired pupil.

To sign or not to sign, that is the question?

There have been long arguments about the best way to communicate and teach the deaf. Obviously, oral communication is the most desirable but not always possible with severely hearing-impaired children. The most vital need is to communicate as fully as possible with the child and it is possible that a rigid approach which only allows oral communication or only signing does not realize the child's potential. The modern concept is total communication which gives the child the opportunity of using all forms of communication to extend language, including speech, formalized gestures, finger spelling, lip reading, and writing.

Finger spelling

In this method, 26 hand positions represent the 26 letters of the English alphabet. This is a slow method of communication.

British sign language

This is used mainly by the deaf adult population; it incorporates both national signs and regional variations and is recognized as a language in its own right.

Signed English

This represents the English language grammatically and also incorporates finger spelling.

Signed supported English

This is simply a method which uses signs for key words to support oral communication.

Cued speech

Different hand shapes close to the speaker's mouth help to differentiate sounds normally invisible with lip reading.

The above gives only a brief description of the manual forms of communication but, as mentioned earlier, the modern concept is to incorporate all different forms of communication (total communication) to give the child as much chance as possible for social integration.

9

GLUE EAR

Glue ear is a descriptive term for the commonest cause of deafness in childhood. The surgical treatment of glue ear is now the most common operation of all performed in children—so much so that one author has described it as 'an epidemic of surgery for glue ear'. No other childhood operation has shown such a dramatic rise in 'popularity' at a time when the overall numbers of operations and hospital admissions for children have declined. At present it is estimated that a million children a year are treated for this condition in the United States, and in England and Wales approximately 50 out of every 10 000 children under the age of ten years will be treated surgically.

WHAT IS GLUE EAR?

Over the years there have been dozens of names, most of which are rather long winded and not particularly accurate, given to describe this condition. Glue ear is in no way a distinct medical term. However, it is very descriptive of the type of fluid found in the middle ear space (which should be filled with air, not fluid), and which lies deep to the ear-drum and connects to the nose via the Eustachian tube (Chapter 2). If one likens this space to a musical drum it will be appreciated that by filling it with fluid the transmission of sound will be severely reduced. The degree of deafness that occurs is much the same as occurs to a normal-hearing person when he places a finger in each ear-canal. The result is that sound can be heard but a good deal of concentration is needed to listen. Many children with this condition will simply switch off, go into a dream world, and fail to progress educationally.

WHY DOES GLUE EAR OCCUR?

Strangely, despite an enormous amount of research, there is still no definite answer to why glue ear occurs in children. There is no doubt that the Eustachian tube is of prime importance in the causation of this condition. Evidence for this comes from children born with a cleft palate, in which the two halves of the roof of the mouth fail to fuse together during development, leaving a midline gap. The back part of the roof of the mouth is soft and forms the soft palate. There are muscles in the soft palate that are normally joined together down the middle, but in the child with cleft palate this may not occur. These muscles are connected to the Eustachian tubes and are in fact the only means by which the Eustachian tube can open. Because this is not possible in the child with cleft palate, owing to lack of anchorage of one muscle to the other, the Eustachian tube remains shut. As was mentioned above, the middle ear space should contain air. This is replenished every time we swallow—the Eustachian tubes open during this movement, allowing air from the back of the nose to go up into the middle ear space. In the child with cleft palate the Eustachian tubes cannot open; therefore air is not replaced with each swallow and fluid (glue) accumulates instead. It is estimated that 90 per cent of one-year-old children with cleft palate have coexisting glue ear.

Non-opening or blockage of the Eustachian tube results in a negative pressure in the middle ear space; this sucks fluid out of the membranes lining the space. If this process continues the lining actually changes its character to become mucus producing, hence the term 'glue ear'. However, glue ear is common and cleft palates are relatively rare. Therefore there must be other reasons for blockage of the

Eustachian tube. One might be adenoid enlargement. The adenoids arise in the back of the nose and may obstruct the opening of the Eustachian tube. Infection from the sinuses and adenoids, or allergy, can cause swelling and blockage of the entrance to the tube.

Another suggestion as to the cause of glue ear is the misuse of antibiotics. Because antibiotics are so effective in relieving the pain of acute infection of the ear, people may often be tempted not to complete the full course of the drug and stop using it after 2 or 3 days when the symptoms have disappeared, instead of continuing it for at least a week. It is possible that although the bacteria are killed, sterile pus remains behind in the middle ear, which itself may cause glue ear.

Whatever the cause, it seems that in most cases the glue is actually produced by abnormal mucus-secreting glands lining the middle ear space. These glands will disappear only if air is allowed to flow into the middle ear space. Encouraging air into the middle ear space is a problem since the glue is too sticky to run back down the tube into the nose, and this is necessary if air is to reach the middle ear. Aeration can be achieved by the myringotomy and grommet (ventilation tube) operation (see below).

IS GLUE EAR A NEW DISEASE?

Most young adults will not have been aware of glue ear when they were children. There seems to have been an explosion of the disease in the last 10–15 years; but it is difficult to know whether there has been a true increase in the incidence or whether it is now just better recognized and judged of more importance than it was in the past. In 1853 Sir William Wilde, father of Oscar Wilde and a distinguished ENT surgeon in Dublin, published a large number of his cases, many of which from his beautiful description were undoubtedly cases of glue ear. Strangely, the literature is then very sparse as regards glue ear cases until 1940 when further reports become available. The main reason that it now seems such a common disease is the excellence of the hearing screening programme which is routine for all five-year-old children and, in many areas, younger children as well.

WHY TREAT GLUE EAR?

Although it is true that many cases of glue ear, if left untreated, will eventually resolve spontaneously, this process may take a matter of years rather than months. The lack of hearing during that time can pose a serious *educational* handicap. It is probably this effect that is the main reason nowadays for suggesting that treatment is worth while and necessary.

Although, in most cases, children do not have any formal schooling before the age of five years, learning is taking place all the time. Even at nursery school, teachers who are aware of the problem will be able to spot the child with glue ear quite easily. Typically, they do not concentrate on one task at a time, and they fidget when the morning story is being read, often gazing out of the window, simply because they cannot hear and have given up bothering to listen. The slightly older child may well be constantly in a dream world and doing 'his own thing' rather than joining in with the rest of the class. In the playground they may appear isolated. There is plenty of evidence that this condition reduces educational attainment and it is perfectly possible that 20 or so years ago many of the 'dunces' in the class were in fact not daft but deaf. The difficulty is that once the child is behind educationally it is a great problem for him to catch up and he may, in fact, never do so. It is unfortunate that children do not seem to recognize the fact that they may be deaf themselves. This is probably because of the slow, insidious onset of the condition.

In the very young child glue ear may also impair *speech and language* development. It is unlikely to cause gross abnormalities of speech since the sound received by the child is not distorted, but only at a much quieter volume. Language delay, however, may be a significant problem. Some parents assume that if their children were deaf they would shout rather than talk at a normal volume. This is true only in the case of inner ear (sensorineural) deafness, where the child cannot monitor his own voice because transmission of sound through the skull is reduced. In glue ear, however, there is nothing wrong with the inner ear. So sound travels readily through the skull and therefore the child has feedback of his own voice, allowing him to regulate the volume of speech. This can be demonstrated by putting your fingers in your own ears and then speaking. Your voice should seem louder than it did with the ears unplugged. This may be the reason why some children with glue ear speak softly, since they assume they are shouting.

The *behaviour* of young children may well also be affected by glue ear. This is difficult to prove, but frustration does build up at not being able to hear properly which may lead to isolation and sometimes aggression. The keen pupil will have had to concentrate very hard during the day and may be grumpy and miserable at home because of the increased efforts he is making at school.

Infection quite frequently occurs and this may be one of the reasons for the child presenting to the doctor. The glue is rich in protein, which is a good culture medium for any bacteria that can reach and feed on it. Repeated episodes of acute ear infections following colds may be caused by re-infection of residual glue in the middle ear.

The final reason for treating glue ear is that occasionally serious *ear-drum damage* occurs. One possibility is that infection may well rupture the ear-drum, leaving a *perforation*. The vast majority of childhood perforations heal, but if the infections are repeated the ear-drum may become weak and eventually a permanent perforation may result. A more serious complication, however, is the occasional association with a serious mastoid disease called *cholesteatoma*. This is probably the result of the pressure of glue causing degeneration of part of the ear-drum, so that it becomes very thin and floppy. This floppy segment may then get drawn into the roof of the middle ear and result in cholesteatoma (see Chapter 11).

Were it not for the above problems it might be justifiable simply to give children hearing aids until their glue ear resolved. However, for the above reasons and from a cosmetic point of view as well this is not readily acceptable.

HOW CAN GLUE EAR BE IDENTIFIED?

Public awareness that this condition is common in children will hopefully increase parental suspicion that something might be wrong with their child rather than assuming that all children say 'eh' and want the television volume turned full on. These are two common symptoms which at present often fail to raise suspicion on the part of the parent.

As described in Chapter 5, the development of speech and language should be a fairly steady and regular process and any deviation from this norm should be regarded by parents as an indication to seek professional advice. Repeated attacks of acute infection is another symptom that might alert parents. The child will usually be taken to the general practitioner and examination of the ears in between attacks may identify glue ear. As mentioned before, behavioural abnormalities may occur but, because there are many other causes of abnormal behaviour in young children, it is unlikely these will be thought of as being due to hearing loss. The greatest advance in identification has been routine hearing testing in the preschool and school age child. Distraction tests and free-field audiometry have been described in an earlier chapter, and pure-tone audiometry is usually possible in the 5-year-old child. The other device which is of great importance in the diagnosis of this condition is tympanometry (see Chapter 3), which measures ear-drum movements with an automatic probe placed in the ear-canal. It does not rely on the child's co-operation but does require the ear-canal to be free of wax. For this reason it is not yet a useful mass screening tool since false readings will occur if the ear-canal has not been cleaned out beforehand. The ideal screening instrument is one that can be used by a wide variety of personnel without the need for specialist back-up. However, a combination of tympanometry and audiometry will pick up nearly all cases of glue ear in the 5-year-old population and is also successful in the preschool child. The characteristic flat trace (Fig. 8) is classical of glue ear. If the child fails these tests he or she is usually retested in a month or so, and if this test is also below par then referral to the patient's family doctor is undertaken. The latter will most probably refer the child to the specialist at the hospital, who will confirm whether or not glue ear is present and whether treatment should be undertaken.

HOW CAN GLUE EAR BE TREATED?

Occasionally no treatment at all is required, since natural fluctuations from normal may occur depending on the age of the child and the season of the year. The older the child, the more likely spontaneous resolution is to occur, simply because with age the skull increases in size and the Eustachian tube becomes more adult sized. It is in fact quite rare to see a child over the age of eight years presenting for the first time with glue ear. Similarly, the condition is undoubtedly worse during the winter months. If a child presents in late spring there is a chance that through the summer, with the absence of colds, the nose will have a period of normality; at this time the Eustachian tube can open and ventilate the middle ears. If initial hearing tests at this time of year show a fairly mild condition, the specialist will often recommend waiting until the beginning of the winter, when the situation will be reviewed. If at this stage glue is still present, then there is much less chance of resolution during the winter months; to avoid further educational delay, treatment will then need to be instituted.

Medical treatment

Unfortunately, medical treatment is not particularly successful. Drugs which contain either antihistamines or adrenaline-like compounds, or a combination of the two are the basis of medical treatment. These drugs reduce congestion in the nose, and so hopefully allow ventilation of the middle ear. The problem with them is that they need to be given for up to six weeks' duration and may have side effects such as making children rather sleepy, or grumpy. It is also very difficult to know whether the drugs are working or whether any improvement taking place is natural. Another group of drugs is available that thins the glue in the middle ear space. Various nasal exercises are occasionally recommended. These include blowing carnival squeakers or balloons with the nose to increase the pressure at the back of the nose and inflate the Eustachian tube and middle ear. However, by far the most common treatment, if treatment is necessary, is surgery.

Surgical treatment

As mentioned above, the most vital feature in curing glue ear is to allow air to reach the middle ear space. This is the basis of the *grommet* (Plate VIII) or *ventilating tube* as it is known in the USA, where about a million such tubes are inserted each year. Before describing the operation of grommet insertion, it should be said that some surgeons believe it important to try to improve nasal function and like to remove any obvious cause of blockage of the Eustachian tube. From a practical point of view, this may mean removal of the adenoids or washing out of the sinuses to help clear infection. However, because grommet insertion can be carried out as a day case, as opposed to the adenoid operation, which requires an overnight stay in hospital, and because there is no definite evidence that removing adenoids helps the eventual resolution of glue ear, more and more surgeons are simply inserting grommets. This is undoubtedly less traumatic to the child, both in terms of discomfort and the length of hospitalization.

The grommet (ventilating tube) operation

In children this operation needs to be done under general anaesthetic. This means a day case admission to a children's ward in a hospital. Most anaesthetists agree that children should be deprived of food and drink for at least six hours before the time of operation. Depending on the anaesthetist, a sedative drug may or may not be given before the child is taken to the operating room. Generally, a tiny needle is placed into a vein on the back of the hand through which a rapidly acting anaesthetic agent is then injected. Once the child is asleep anaesthesia is usually maintained by supplying an anaesthetic gas through a face-mask.

The surgeon will examine the ear using an operating microscope and clean out any small pieces of wax that might be obscuring the view of the ear-drum. A tiny slit is made in the ear-drum with a very fine knife. This is called a *myringotomy* (Fig. 12a). Through this fine slit in the ear-drum a tiny suction tube is used to vacuum out the sticky middle ear fluid (glue). Usually it is possible to extract all the glue; once this has been accomplished the grommet is inserted through the same slit (Fig. 12b). Both ears are normally operated on and the child recovers very quickly once the anaesthetic agents are removed. It is unusual for there to be any pain and most parents will notice a significant improvement in the child's hearing within the first 24 hours. Within a week the ear-drum is well healed around the grommet.

The length of time that a grommet will stay in place varies, depending on its design. The most basic type usually lasts

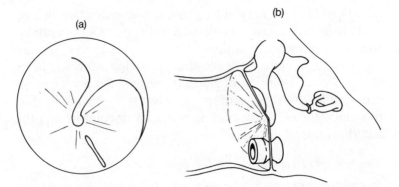

Fig. 12 (a) Incision in ear-drum (myringotomy) prior to insertion of grommet. **(b)** Grommet in ear-drum.

about six months and is rejected from the ear-drum into the ear-canal where it gradually migrates to the outside. Because it is so tiny, it will then often be lost. In nearly all cases, the ear-drum heals quite spontaneously once the grommet has been rejected and perforations are rare. Regular follow-up while grommets are in place is sensible; it is also important to check the hearing after rejection of a grommet to make sure there is no recurrence of glue. About 80 per cent of children are cured with only one set of grommets; however, in 20 per cent of cases further grommets may be necessary until either nature or ageing of the child cures the glue ear. The object, as has been mentioned before, is to keep the child hearing normally until he has outgrown the problem.

A frequently asked question is 'can my child go swimming with grommets?' For the first week after a grommet has been inserted it is suggested that no water be allowed in the ear-canal. A simple ear-plug for use when hair washing and bathing is cotton wool dipped in petroleum jelly and placed in the outer ear-canal. It is very unlikely that splashes of water from swimming, even if the head is momentarily put beneath the surface of the water, will actually run through the tiny hole in the grommet. This is because the surface tension of water is such that it will not flow down the narrow channel in the grommet. However, diving should be banned since the increased pressure could well force water through the grommet into the middle ear and possibly set up infection. If infection does occur, either through swimming or through a normal middle ear infection, the child very rarely complains of pain since there is no build-up of infection and pressure within the middle ear space; the pus simply leaks out of the grommet to appear as a messy discharge in the ear canal. If this occurs it is treated with antibiotics, usually given orally. Occasionally, because the grommet acts as a foreign body, the discharge continues. If it does not settle easily with antibiotics given orally, then antibiotic ear-drops can be most effective.

The most common complication of grommet insertion is scarring of the ear-drum; this occurs in about 20–40 per cent of cases. It is most likely to occur if repeated grommets are necessary. Luckily, there is very little evidence that this interferes at all with normal hearing and it simply remains as a blemish on the ear-drum. This is visible only to a doctor examining the ear and is of no particular medical importance.

The long term outlook for a child who has had glue ear and grommet operations is excellent; most patients can look forward to normal hearing. The incidence of adult forms of chronic infective deafness appears to be falling owing to better care of the childhood problem of glue ear.

It seems that glue is here to stay and for the present grommets (ventilating tubes) will continue to be necessary. A glue thinning and draining drug might hopefully be available in future, but until it is we must all look out for hearing loss in children caused by glue ear to prevent the educational and other problems detailed in this chapter.

Part II

ADULT PROBLEMS

10

WAX

Wax deserves a separate chapter as it is the most common self-diagnosis of the cause of hearing loss and a frequent reason for referral for medical attention. Although wax impaction can give rise to hearing impairment, which of course is simple to correct, sadly it is not usually the sole cause. However, someone with an already established hearing loss who then experiences increased difficulty may well be restored to their former state by the removal of wax.

WHY DO WE HAVE WAX?

Wax is produced by tiny glands in the outer third of the skin of the ear-canal. It is actually secreted as tiny, white droplets which, if left undisturbed, turn to a sticky fluid. They gradually become yellow or brown with exposure to air to give the characteristic appearance of normal wax. It is a normal constituent of our ear-canals but is absent in some diseased states, notably inflammation of the ear-canal (*external otitis*). Recovery from this painful condition is often heralded by the re-appearance of wax in the ear-canal. An absence of wax is thus associated with infection, which therefore presupposes it has a protective function for the ear-canal.

Wax collects in the outer third of the ear-canal to provide a chemical barrier to infection and a physical obstruction to foreign bodies, such as dust, that might otherwise accumulate in it. The chemical nature of the barrier is that the wax is acidic and contains a high concentration of lipids (fats), which serves to make the skin of the ear-canal waterproof. This prevents moisture, for example in hot, sticky climates or after showers, macerating the skin lining or entering the hair follicles, thereby causing infection. Enzymes and immunoglobulins have also been discovered, possibly adding to the anti-infective role of wax.

The amount of wax varies enormously between people and there seems no obvious explanation for this. Some people consider wax to be a sign of uncleanliness and spend a good deal of time carefully cleaning their own and their childrens' ear-canals. However, removal of wax eliminates the barrier to infection and the trauma caused by removal, even with soft cotton buds, may well predispose to ear infection. Some will also tend to try and flush the wax from their ears using modified syringes; however, this dissolves the greasy, protective lining and again will predipose to infection. Soapy water in the ear-canal changes the pH (acidity level) to an alkaline state, which again removes the natural bacterial and fungal barrier to infection.

SYMPTOMS

There is no doubt that wax does cause symptoms, the most usual being deafness and sometimes slight discomfort. Deafness does not, however, occur while there is even the minutest gap for the sound to get past the wax to reach the ear-drum. It is often precipitated by a small amount of water going into the ear-canal, for instance from swimming, which simply moves the wax a bit or causes it to swell slightly and block the canal completely.

TREATMENT

Ears are best left alone and, provided that the wax is causing no symptoms, it should not be disturbed. The usual method of removing wax is by the use of an ear-syringe. This needs to be done carefully by experienced personnel since high pressure, fine water jets can damage the ear-drum. There are many proprietary preparations on the market for dissolving wax, some of which cause irritation if there is any associated infection. Simple remedies include sodium bicarbonate solution, which, although an alkali, is an effective way of breaking down impacted wax. The use of simple olive oil or liquid paraffin may help to soften the wax, and hydrogen peroxide mixed with a sterile oil is also an effective way of releasing wax.

If the patient has an underlying perforation of the ear-drum, then syringeing should not be used, nor should ear-drops be employed. Help from an ear specialist is the only solution. He will probably remove the wax with special wax hooks or use a vacuum suction apparatus.

Wax should be regarded as a normal feature and on the whole is best left alone.

11

HEARING LOSS DUE TO INFECTION

Apart from otosclerosis (see Chapter 12), most adult middle ear problems are secondary to infection. Many of these probably arise in childhood; however, they are included in the adult section of this book since it is often better to wait until adult life to correct them.

PERFORATIONS OF THE EAR-DRUM

The medical profession divides perforations of the ear-drum into two types—'safe' and 'unsafe'. 'Safe' perforations occur in the lower half of the ear-drum, whereas 'unsafe' perforations occur in the upper half (Fig. 13). Luckily, the 'unsafe' variety are rare, but are associated with complications because of their association with the disease called *cholesteatoma*, which extends into the mastoid bone.

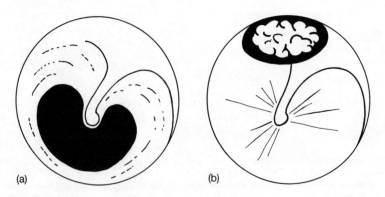

Fig. 13 The two types of perforation: **(a)** 'safe', and **(b)** 'unsafe'.

'Safe' perforations

'Safe' perforations most usually are either secondary to infection via the Eustachian tube or due to trauma. Recurrent infections in childhood may lead to a perforated ear-drum; although this normally heals after each infection has abated, it occasionally does not, becoming a permanent perforation with associated middle ear deafness and recurrent discharge.

Trauma to the ear-drum may occur through poking objects into the ear-canal or from blast injuries. All manner of foreign bodies causing injury to the ear-drum have been recorded, and quite often this is associated with the patient trying to clean wax out of his own ears or giving them a bit of a scratch with a matchstick or similar object. This is not recommended! The author has even seen a boy who was dressing up as an Indian chief come into hospital because his little sister thought he would look smarter with feathers coming out of his ears and she had rammed the quills through both tympanic membranes! Children are notoriously interested in their various orifices and the ear is one where serious damage can occur if it is abused.

Blast injuries from explosion or being hit over the ear-canal may lead to rupture through pressure waves momentarily increasing the air pressure in the external ear and resulting in rupture of the only movable structure—the ear-drum. The practice of cuffing an errant child over his ears is dangerous!

Symptoms

A middle ear deafness will occur with all except the smallest of perforations. The degree of hearing loss will depend on the size although, provided the middle ear ossicles are intact, it is rarely more than 35 dB (Fig. 14).

Discharge from the ear-canal is commonly associated with perforations and will often be recurrent unless the cause of the infection is uncovered and cured. Recurrent infections

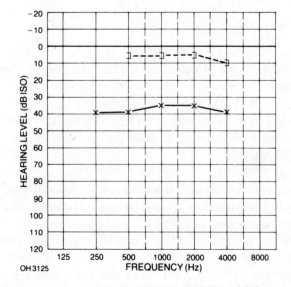

OH 3125

Fig. 14 Pure-tone audiogram showing 35 dB middle ear hearing loss associated with an ear-drum perforation.

arise either because of nasal sepsis from sinuses, adenoids, etc. creeping up the Eustachian tube to the middle ear and leaking out through the perforation, or occasionally through infection from the mastoid bone. The mastoid (Chapter 2) is really an extension of the middle ear cavity; it is a honeycomb of cells normally containing air like the middle ear and is connected via a small passage to the roof of the middle ear. The mastoid bone can be felt as a hard bulge behind the ear. In recurrent middle ear infection the honeycomb in the mastoid may become full of chronic infection and act as a reservoir, spilling over into the middle ear, and causing it to leak through the perforation. Often X-rays are suggested to assess the state of the mastoid honeycomb of air cells.

Treatment

Medical. Medical treatment, after a hunt for the cause of the recurrent discharge, may mean antibiotics to eradicate infection from the adenoids, sinuses, or mastoid air cells. It will not, however, close the perforation once it is established.

Surgical. These perforations are called 'safe' because no serious harm will come to the patient by not having treatment. Surgery is often the patient's choice—for example he would like his hearing improved, to go swimming (a perforation means that the ear is no longer waterproof and would allow water to enter the ear, causing recurrent discharge), to join the armed forces, or to be rid of recurrent discharge.

Surgical treatment involves closing the perforation. A delicate microsurgical technique called *Myringoplasty* is often done via the ear-canal and usually under a general anaesthetic. A patch is placed over the perforation to heal it (Fig. 15). The repair patch is usually obtained from the patient's own tissue—from the layer of tough fibrous tissue (*temporalis fascia*) which covers one of the muscles in the scalp immediately above the ear. The patch or graft is normally kept in place by careful positioning and dressings in the ear-canal. These dressings are usually removed about three weeks after the operation, by which time the graft will hopefully have 'taken'. Aftercare is a matter of keeping water out of the ear until it has healed properly and avoiding sudden pressure changes (such as from blowing the nose hard, diving, or flying) since severe fluctuations in middle ear

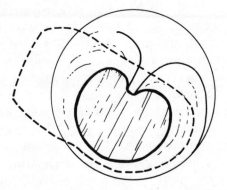

Fig. 15 Myringoplasty—patch placed across the perforation.

pressure may cause the graft to become detached. Hard nose blowing is probably safe after about six weeks and flying and diving are best avoided for three months after the dressings are removed. Successful grafting occurs in over 80 per cent of cases.

'Unsafe' perforations

Luckily, the 'unsafe' type of perforation is rarer but is associated with the disease *cholesteatoma*. The perforation is in the upper part of the ear-drum (Fig. 13b) and involves the mastoid bone A characteristic of cholesteatoma is the destruction of bone; this damages the middle ear ossicles and, more significantly, the balance organ or semicircular canals (*labyrinth*) (see Fig. 1) and bony covering to the facial nerve, which can result in facial paralysis. These perforations are called 'unsafe' because of such bone-damaging properties and their potential to erode from the mastoid into more serious areas such as the brain. Fortunately, all these complications are rare and can be avoided if the disease is spotted in time. Cholesteatoma usually presents when it becomes infected and the discharge from the ear has the very distinct characteristic feature of being extremely smelly. The safe perforations described before may discharge but smell is a rarity; therefore an offensive discharge should always be taken seriously.

The treatment is not medical but surgical and one of various forms of mastoid operations will be required to eradicate the disease. Hearing conservation or reconstruction is, unfortunately, of secondary importance to clearing the disease because of its potential danger to the patient. Most modern surgeons will, however, want eventually to reconstruct the hearing and the operations are often 'staged' —the first stage to eradicate the disease and the second to reconstruct the middle ear hearing mechanism.

Unfortunately, most types of mastoid operation required for cholesteatoma result in what is referred to as a 'mastoid cavity'. Instead of the ear-canal leading straight down to the ear-drum it is also linked with the inside of the mastoid bone. This means that wax and debris build up in this large potential space and the patient needs regular care, usually annually, by an ENT specialist to clean the cavity. Although 20 per cent of these cavities discharge intermittently, they are usually safe. Discharge is, however, a nuisance for the patient with a mastoid cavity and revision surgery to stop the leakage is commonly recommended.

DAMAGE TO THE OSSICULAR CHAIN

As was mentioned in Chapter 2, the three ossicles are very delicate and infection or trauma can damage the connections between them. The thin strut of the incus where it joins the stapes is particularly vulnerable. It has a poor blood supply and if this is damaged through infection it simply rots away (Fig. 16a). This results in a breakdown of sound transmission

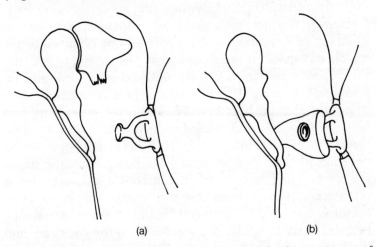

(a)   (b)

Fig. 16 (a) Ossicular disruption—erosion of the long process of the incus which is no longer in contact with the stapes. **(b)** Damaged incus removed and reshaped to fit as a connection between the malleus and stapes.

from the tympanic membrane to the inner ear; whereas a perforation on its own results in only a 30 dB deafness, discontinuity of the ossicles often results in a 50 dB hearing loss. Indeed, the clinician diagnosing a perforation will suspect ossicular problems as well if the deafness is more than 30 dB. Although discontinuity of the junction between the incus and the stapes is the commonest cause, all other combinations are possible. In mastoid surgery for cholesteatoma it is often necessary to remove some of the ossicles to clear the disease.

Repair presents an interesting surgical challenge for the surgeon, one where modern microsurgery comes into its own and opens up huge possibilities for inventiveness to repair the defect. Without a doubt, the best results come from using the patient's own damaged ossicles for repair, but occasionally there are none spare and plastic materials or even transplanted bone or cartilage is used.

For interest, two possibilities are described. These operations are usually performed down the ear-canal using an operating microscope. Assuming the ear-drum is not perforated or has not been previously repaired, part of it is lifted out of its seating so that access can be obtained to the middle ear space. If the incus and stapes are out of contact, the patient's own incus can be removed, reshaped, and repositioned as in Fig. 16b. Special glues are occasionally used to hold the repair together. The ear-drum is replaced and held by packing until healed, which usually takes about three or four days, after which the hearing will hopefully be noticeably better. A more tricky situation is when the stapes superstructure (the arch of the stirrup) is missing; this is often accompanied by an absent incus or malleus. A T- or mushroom-shaped piece of cartilage or plastic material may be used to try to bridge the gap between the ear-drum and the footplate of the stapes (Fig. 17).

These are just two of the many ingenious techniques used in this exciting field of middle ear reconstruction. A considerable amount of experimental work is at present going on to

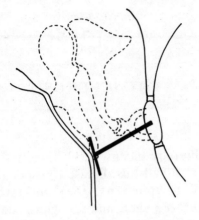

Fig. 17 Artificial prosthesis to connect ear-drum to inner ear in a case of total loss of ossicles.

try to find suitable materials for replacement of the ear-drum and the middle ear ossicles which will not be rejected by the patient, are easy to use, and produce good, reliable hearing results. At the present time, however, nature seems to prefer the body's own materials to plastic or transplanted ones.

12

OTOSCLEROSIS

Otosclerosis literally means 'hardening of the bone of the ear'. The French call this disease 'otospongiosis', which is possibly more accurate since the bone involved tends to become thicker, bloodier, and spongier. The actual process is as follows: abnormal lumps of bone appear in the middle ear around the footplate of the stapes (see Chapter 2), preventing it moving freely in and out of the oval window. This has the effect of stiffening the ossicular chain, leading to a reduction in the conduction of sound from the ear-drum to the inner ear, and giving rise to a middle ear deafness. The surgery for otosclerosis has been one of the most exciting advances in the history of medical science. The modern operation is called *stapedectomy* and has been made possible through developments in microsurgical techniques and the invention of the operating microscope about 30 years ago. The ability to restore hearing to a patient previously rendered very hard of hearing is a most gratifying occurrence for both the patient and surgeon.

HISTORICAL BACKGROUND

This condition has been recognized for well over a hundred years and surgical operations were being performed at the end of the last century, despite the fact that there were no operating microscopes or very fine instruments and only primitive anaesthetics. Since stapedectomy is one of the most delicate of all surgical operations, it is hardly surprising that these early results ended in failure, with often disastrous complications, which resulted in the abandonment of further attempts at surgery for about 50 years. In the late 1930s an operation called 'fenestration' was devised; however, this is no longer performed because the results it gave were very much inferior to the modern stapedectomy operation, which was first performed in 1958. Since that time there have been many modifications and developments in microsurgical techniques, which have improved the success rate of this operation to well over 90 per cent.

A FEW FACTS

This disease occurs only in humans and is rare in negroid races, although it is a relatively common cause of adult middle ear deafness in other races. In the latter, it causes hearing loss in 4 out of 1000 adults; however, some studies based on post-mortem evidence have suggested that up to 10 per cent of the population are affected.

Most commonly, the condition presents between the age of 20 and 30 years and seems to be twice as common in women as in men. This is probably a falsely high bias towards women for two reasons. First, it occurs more frequently on one side only in men; so it is therefore less of a handicap and less likely to cause that person to seek help. Secondly, the disease appears to accelerate during the latter part of pregnancy, often bringing the woman to the attention of the ear specialist. It is a genetically determined disease and in 70 per cent of patients other members of the family with the disease can be traced.

Although the condition usually presents between 20 and 30 years of age, there is in the vast majority of cases a steady progression of hearing loss from the age of 20 and if untreated a very severe deafness is likely to be present after about 30 years. About 10 per cent of patients seem to level out at a 50 dB loss; however, the other 90 per cent eventually become much worse than this. Another feature is that not only is the middle ear affected (conductive deafness), but with time an inner ear deafness also occurs. The latter condition is untreatable. It is reasonable to say therefore that, prior to the advent of the modern operation of stapedectomy, the patient would most probably be doomed to a life of severe deafness by the age of 60.

SYMPTOMS AND SIGNS OF OTOSCLEROSIS

By far the commonest symptom is the complaint of hearing loss. As mentioned before, this is usually in both ears, although about 20 per cent of men are affected in one ear only. Apart from hearing loss, which may have been noticed in pregnancy, quite a common feature is the ability to hear better in noisy surroundings. This is probably because the speaker has to raise his voice against the background noise to levels above the threshold of the sufferer's hearing loss. Sometimes tinnitus, and more rarely giddiness, are also complained of.

When the specialist examines the ear he will usually remark that the ear-drum looks completely normal and yet in simple tuning fork tests (as described in Chapter 3) the patient will hear better when the fork is applied to the bone behind the ear than when it is held in front of the ear. This will tell the doctor that there is failure of conduction between the ear-drum and inner ear. Since the former is normal, the problem is most likely to be due to one of the three bones in the middle ear; fixation of the stapes by otosclerosis is the most likely diagnosis even at this early stage. Figure 18 shows a typical audiogram. A further confirmatory test is called the *stapedial reflex*. This is an interesting test and is carried out using the equipment described under tympanometry in Chapter 3. It relies on the fact that the stapes bone has a small tendon attached to it which has the ability to tighten in response to loud noise.

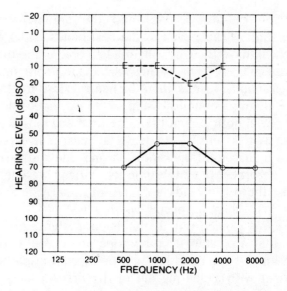

Fig. 18 Pure-tone audiogram showing the typical middle ear deafness of otosclerosis.

The application of a loud sound, usually over 80 dB, will cause the tendon to twitch and the slight movement of the stapes causes a corresponding movement of the ear-drum which can be measured with the tympanometer. If the stapes is fixed by otosclerosis, then no matter how hard the tendon twitches there will be no movement of the stapes and no movement of the ear-drum; therefore an absent stapedial reflex is likely to be present in otosclerosis. Once these tests have been carried out, a fairly confident diagnosis of otosclerosis can be made and treatment can then be discussed with the patient.

MANAGEMENT OF OTOSCLEROSIS

The choice of treatment is between the provision of a hearing aid and operation (stapedectomy). The argument against the provision of a hearing aid is that it will not prevent progression of the disease, and the argument against stapedectomy is that, even in the best hands, 2 per cent of patients will have their hearing made worse in the operated ear by the surgery. This is due to damage to the inner ear and occasionally results in total hearing loss in that ear. Because of this possibility, stapedectomy should never be carried out in both ears at the same time and most surgeons agree that it is sensible to leave at least a five-year gap between a successful operation on one side and carrying it out on the other. If by the time the patient presents to the specialist there is already a degree of underlying inner ear hearing loss, then a special hearing test called a *speech audiogram* is carried out. If this is poor, then there is less chance that the stapedectomy operation will make the hearing much better and it might be more sensible to treat the patient with a hearing aid in the first instance. Many specialists consider that it is worth giving the patient a trial with a hearing aid anyway, since if the aid is effective it is often the case that an operation will be as well. In those patients who have the disease in only one ear, surgery can still be useful in balancing up the hearing for directional perception of sound. Finally, it is usual to wait until the disease is out of its active phase, which means not operating in teenagers and delaying until further pregnancies are no longer considered. If a hearing aid is the choice then, because the audiogram reveals a fairly flat type of hearing loss, a straightforward, behind-the-ear, or in-the-ear hearing aid can be supplied with every hope of a good result.

Stapedectomy

This operation is one of the most satisfying operations to perform. However, it is an exceedingly delicate operation requiring a great deal of skill and absolute sterility. Because of the slight risk of damaging the hearing from the surgery, the poorer-hearing ear is chosen. The operation can be performed under local, but more usually general, anaesthesia, and is carried out using an operating microscope for vision down the ear-canal. Using micro-instruments, the ear-drum is lifted from its bed and reflected forwards to give access to the contents of the middle ear (Fig. 19a). It is only at this stage that the diagnosis can be confirmed and this is done simply by gently moving the stapes to see whether it is indeed fixed (Fig. 19b). Having divided the tendon, the stapes superstructure is then removed. This leaves the footplate of the stapes fixed rigidly in the oval window and a small hole is very gently drilled through this footplate. At this moment, extreme precision is necessary since there is only about 0.4 mm between the footplate and the delicate inner ear structures. A false stapes (prosthesis), which is normally shaped like a shepherd's crook (Plate IX), is clipped over the incus with the other end just entering the hole drilled in the footplate (Fig. 19c). The chain of bones is now intact and mobile and when the ear-drum is moved this movement is transmitted once again into the inner ear, but this time via the prosthesis. The ear-drum is now simply replaced and a small piece of dressing inserted into the ear-canal while healing takes place. These dressings are usually removed within a week when, in most patients, there is already a gratifying gain of hearing. There is occasionally slight dizziness on moving the head after the operation, but this usually settles within 48 hours. Healing is complete by about 2 weeks and 90 per cent of patients are delighted with the result, although if there has been some inner ear hearing loss as well it will be impossible to restore the hearing to absolute normality. Hospitalization for two or three days is usually necessary.

The operation often seems miraculous to the patient. Even in those in whom a near-total deafness was present before the operation, about 50 per cent will be able to hear quite effectively with the help of a hearing aid, which would not have previously been possible.

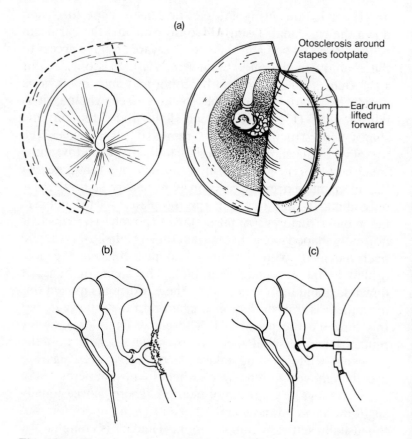

Fig. 19(a) First stage in stapedectomy: **(left)** an incision is made (shown by the dotted line); **(right)** the ear-drum is carefully lifted from its seating and rolled forward to give access to the middle ear. **Fig. 19(b)** The stapes fixed in the oval window by otosclerotic bone. **Fig. 19(c)** The Stapes arch is removed and replaced by a prosthesis—the crook is attached to the incus and the other end is in a small hole drilled in the fixed footplate. Transmission of sound to the inner ear can now take place.

SUMMARY

Thirty years have elapsed since the first of the modern generation stapedectomies was performed and this means that we still cannot be perfectly certain what will happen in the long term to young patients who have had these operations, but it certainly seems that without them a steady progression to severe hearing loss would be likely. Occasional severe late deafness occurs in stapedectomized patients and for this reason a note of caution needs to be used before considering surgery on the other ear. Having said that, modern refinements and better training of surgeons continue to make this operation safer.

MENIÈRE'S DISEASE

True Menière's disease is really quite rare; yet many patients referred to ENT specialists with the symptoms of deafness, tinnitus, and dizziness have been labelled as having Menière's disease, a diagnosis which is probably incorrect. For this reason, the subject is given a separate chapter.

Prosper Menière, who worked at the Imperial Institute for Deaf Mutes in Paris, wrote a description in 1861 of the symptoms of Menière's disease which has not been bettered to this day. The problem facing those that treat this disease today is that the pathology is still not truly understood.

SYMPTOMS

The condition classically begins before the age of 50 and usually affects only one ear, that ear having previously been quite healthy. The symptoms include deafness, tinnitus, and dizziness, of which dizziness is by far the most dramatic of the symptoms since it is so prostrating. These attacks come in phases when the patient may be repeatedly very disabled. Remission then occurs, which may last months or years. Eventually, if the attacks persist, the hearing begins to deteriorate permanently.

'Menière's attack'

The classical attack is as follows. First the patient will complain of tinnitus (ringing or buzzing) in one ear followed by a feeling of fullness in that ear. At this stage the hearing appears to become dull and may well be a bit distorted. The tinnitus and dullness in hearing increase and then, apparently without any warning, severe and usually rotatory dizziness occurs with accompanying nausea and vomiting, which frequently forces the patient to take to his or her bed. The dizziness often lasts for 6 hours or so in the acute phase and then leaves the patient feeling wobbly and weak for one or two days. Once the patient has recovered from the vertigo, the tinnitus is often less and the hearing improves. Although this is the classical description, there are many variants and this makes it difficult to be sure of the diagnosis. The attacks may be repeated at weekly intervals and sometimes more frequently for a matter of a month or so, and then apparently die away, only to return again many months later.

If hearing tests are carried out in the remission period they may well show near normal hearing or, more often, a low frequency inner ear deafness. If the hearing is tested at the beginning of the attack the low frequency inner ear deafness is more severe. One of the main features in the diagnosis of this condition is the fluctuating nature of the inner ear deafness. Although middle ear deafness may fluctuate for many reasons, the only likely cause of inner ear fluctuation is Menière's disease. It is therefore important, if the diagnosis is to be made correctly, that the patient should be under the care of a specialist who has facilities for hearing tests.

The gap between attacks may last so long that it seems that the disease has cured itself. More frequently, however, they continue and over the course of time the hearing becomes worse; eventually most end up with a very severe, one-sided hearing loss. Once this has happened, however, the disease seems to burn itself out and the prostrating dizziness is much less of a problem. The sufferer naturally worries that the disease will start up in his remaining good ear but, luckily, this is very uncommon.

PATHOLOGY

Although the symptoms are well described, the pathology is still unclear, for the only abnormal feature that is regularly found is that the membrane of the inner ear is very distended with excess inner ear fluid. It is thought that as the distention occurs the membranes stretch, and the feeling of fullness and increasing hearing loss arise. The prostrating dizziness probably happens at the time that the inner ear membrane ruptures. This allows mixing of the different inner ear fluids, which causes an electrical discharge giving rise to the severe dizziness. The rupture then heals and the patient recovers. The process then begins all over again. The problem is to know whether excess fluid is being produced or whether there is reduced absorption. Whatever the case, the result is the same and treatment is directed to controlling the symptoms, preventing the build-up of fluid, or allowing it to drain away more easily.

TREATMENT

The most important aspect of treatment is undoubtedly strong reassurance that this is a non-fatal condition, that long periods of remission are likely, and that medical treatment will help suppress the symptoms in the vast majority of patients. Surgical treatment is necessary in about 10 per cent of cases and can significantly improve the situation. Therefore a note of optimism is reasonable when counselling patients with this condition.

Acute attack

Usually when there is acute vomiting the only practical treatment is for the patient to go to bed and be given drugs by injection which will suppress the dizziness. Injectable forms of seasick remedies are commonly prescribed.

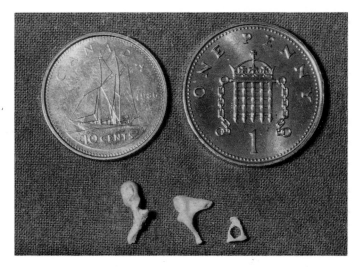

Plate I. Ossicles—malleus (left), incus (centre), and stapes (right) compared in size with ten cents and one penny coins.

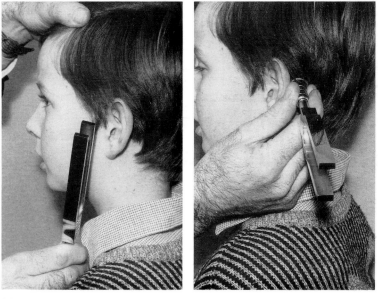

(a)   (b)

Plate II. A child listening to a tuning fork held (a) at the ear canal and (b) behind the ear, to see which is heard louder.

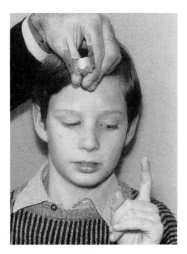

Plate III. Tuning fork held on the centre of the forehead being referred to the apparently better ear.

(a)

(b)

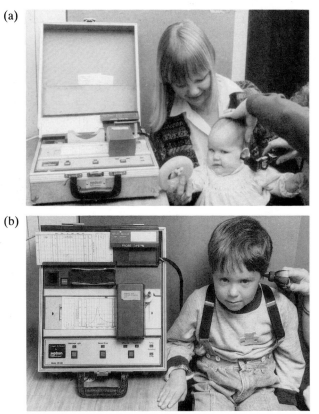

Plate IV. A tympanometer being used with (a) a baby and (b) a young child. An airtight seal is obtained using an auroscope with a tightly fitting ear-piece. Once a seal is obtained the pressure is automatically varied.

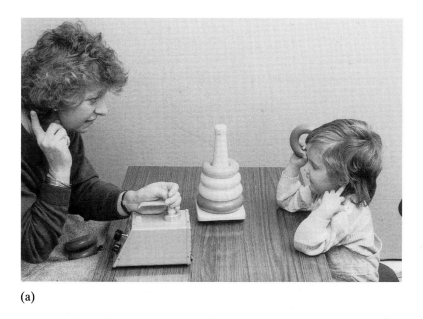

(a)

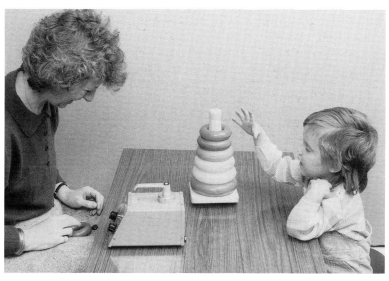

(b)

Plate V (a) and (b). Free-field conditioning audiometry: each time the child hears a tone she puts a ring on the peg.

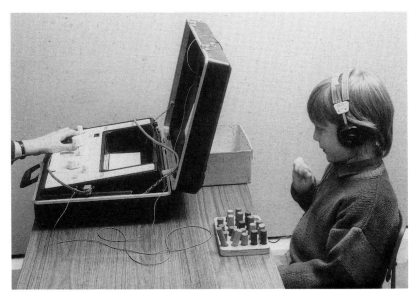

Plate VI. Headphone audiometry for the older child, who puts a block in the box in response to the tone.

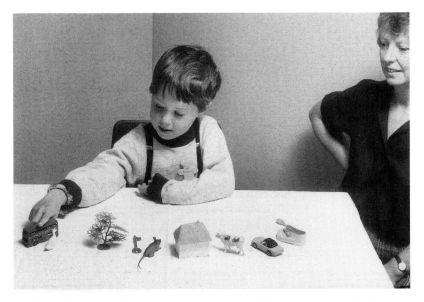

Plate VII. Speech discrimination tests: the child picks up toys which have similar sounding names (e.g. house and mouse) in response to the tester seated behind and to one side.

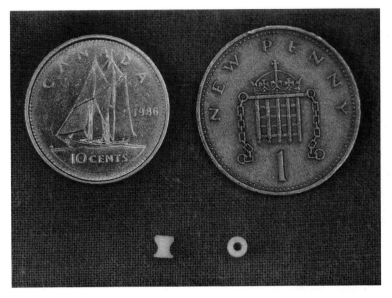

Plate VIII. Commonly used grommet (from side and top view) compared in size with a ten cents and one penny coin.

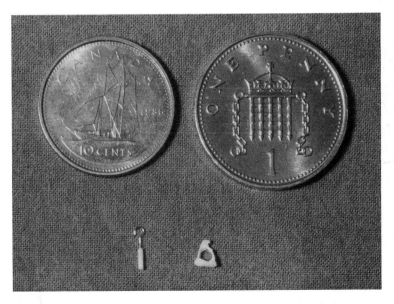

Plate IX. Normal stapes (right) and artificial replacement in relation to ten cents and one penny coins.

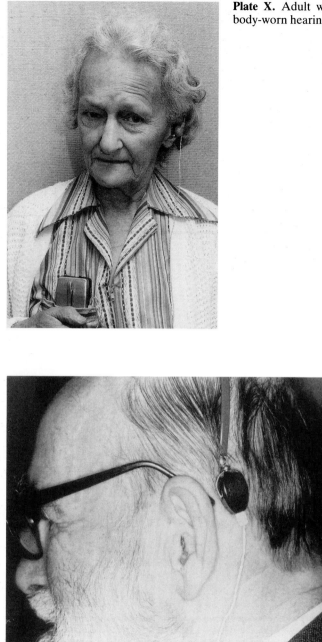

Plate X. Adult wearing body-worn hearing aid.

Plate XI. Adult wearing bone-conducting hearing aid.

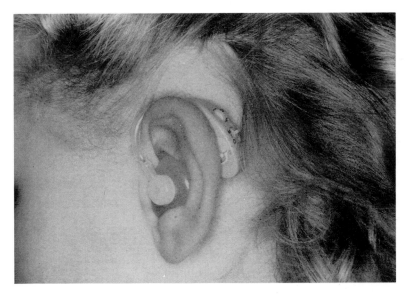

Plate XII. Behind-the-ear hearing aid.

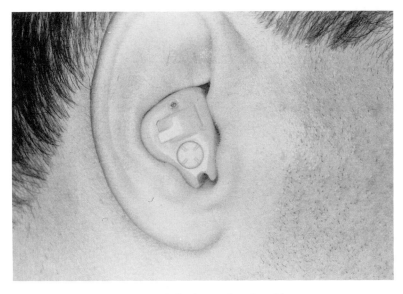

Plate XIII. In-the-ear hearing aid.

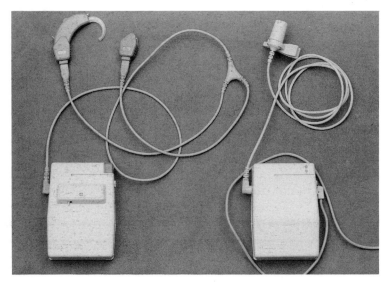

(a)

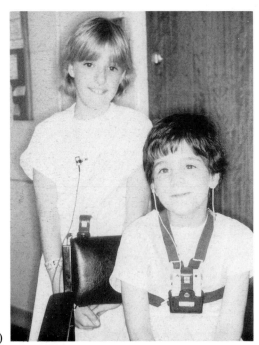

(b)

Plate XIV. Radio hearing aid: (a) the teacher or parent wears the microphone which transmits to the receiver on the child's chest and from there to the amplifier in the post-aural hearing aids; (b) two sisters, one (seated) wearing a radio hearing aid, the other wearing the microphone.

Remission phase

If the disease is completely in remission, there will be no symptoms and probably no need for treatment. The problem with any disease which has long remission phases is that, if treatment is being used, it is very difficult to know whether it is the natural history of the disease or the treatment that brings about the cure.

In order to reduce the excessive fluid within the inner ear, treatment is designed to prevent its build-up or improve drainage once it has occurred. It is suggested that reducing dietary salt, which is quite a powerful fluid retainer, may be helpful. However, there is no scientific evidence for this.

It is felt that the circulation of blood to the inner ear may in some way be defective in Menière's disease, and this causes a build-up of fluid. Drugs are frequently given to improve this blood supply and the most powerful of these is the inhalation of carbon dioxide, as mentioned in Chapter 14 on sudden deafness. However, this is not a practical suggestion during the remission phase of this disease. Other so-called vasodilator drugs are often tried, the most popular one in the UK at present being beta-histine.

The use of diuretics (drugs that increase the amount of fluid excretion in the urine) has also been popular, but there is little evidence that these drugs improve the progress of the disease.

Antihistamines have a useful sedative effect on the inner ear and may control minor bouts of dizziness, but probably do not affect the natural course of the disease. They are, however, the most common type of drug used in travel sickness.

Surgical treatment

If the disease progresses and medical treatment fails to control the frequent disabling attacks of dizziness, then surgery needs to be considered. However, this is usually only required by 10 per cent of patients.

The type of surgery will almost certainly depend on whether the patient has useful functioning hearing in the affected ear. If there is no hearing or it is at such a level that it is completely useless, then the most suitable operation is normally the complete destruction of the inner ear. This is called *labyrinthectomy* and effectively destroys the inner ear membranes. Obviously, the patient is left without hearing, but the vertigo is nearly always controlled very successfully, though tinnitus may well persist.

If the hearing is functional, there is a reluctance to destroy it surgically, and other hearing-preserving procedures have been designed. At present the most common operation is *saccus endolymphatic drainage*. The saccus endolymphaticus is a little out-pouching of the inner ear membrane. When identified, it can be opened and the theory is that as the fluid in the inner ear builds up it simply leaks out of this opening into the mastoid bone. It is difficult to assess accurately the results of this operation, but it can be very favourable in reducing dizziness without damaging hearing. Once again the results on tinnitus are very unpredictable.

It is also possible to cut the nerve of balance (*vestibular nerve*) as it goes into the brain. This, however, is a major neurosurgical operation and there is a risk of damaging the auditory nerve as well.

There are a number of other operations which are beyond the scope of this book, but it should be remembered that in conditions where the pathology is ill-understood and where the nature of the disease has the capacity to remit completely, the assessment of treatment, whether medical or surgical, is very difficult. It is the author's belief that strong reassurance with medical control of the symptoms, especially vertigo, is the most useful management for the majority of cases. Surgical destruction of the inner ear is reserved for those with poor or absent hearing and severe, recurrent, prostrating dizziness.

14

SUDDEN HEARING LOSS

Luckily, sudden and apparently unexplained total loss of hearing is extremely rare. Sudden partial loss is, however, quite common and is usually associated with middle ear problems.

MIDDLE EAR

Many people with partial, sudden hearing loss from Eustachian tube obstruction, such as might occur with a cold or on descent in an aircraft, feel that they have suffered a quite catastrophic loss in hearing. In fact they have probably lost only a small fraction of their normal hearing; nevertheless this is very real and sometimes quite frightening. If the patient is elderly and already has natural ageing deafness, a sudden 20 dB increase in hearing loss makes this handicap severe. Fortunately the situation nearly always resolves spontaneously with time—for instance when the cold is better. It may take a few weeks before the person feels their hearing is back to normal. Decongestant nasal sprays and antihistamine tablets can speed resolution by shrinking the lining of the nose and opening the Eustachian tube. This allows pressure to equalize or fluid to drain from the middle ear back into the nose.

SENSORINEURAL (INNER EAR AND NERVE)

These are extremely rare; the problem for the doctor is to remember to consider sensorineural causes of sudden hear-

ing loss when the vast majority of patients come with partial
middle ear loss as just described. It is, however, extremely
important because early treatment may possibly reverse the
hearing loss, whereas this is highly unlikely if three weeks or
more have elapsed from onset to specialist referral. The
sufferer should be able to tell the difference between the two
types, since even with severe middle ear deafness amplified
voices can still be heard and there is no distortion. Sudden
inner ear deafness, however, is usually total. If a loud 'masking' noise is applied to the good ear then nothing or only
very distorted sound can be heard with the affected one. If
this is the case, urgent specialist referral is essential. Luckily
it is almost unheard of for both ears to fail at the same time
whereas sudden, partial middle ear deafness may affect
both.

Possible reasons for sudden sensorineural hearing loss

The word 'possible' is used here since nothing is proved.
Infection from viruses, particularly mumps, measles, and the
shingles virus have been implicated.

Generalized blood vessel disease (atherosclerosis) may
cause damage to the blood supply of the inner ear by furring
up of the tiny blood vessels supplying it. The cells of the
inner ear cannot survive without oxygen and if there is a
deficient blood supply this might well cause inner ear deafness.

Menière's disease (see Chapter 13) may be characterized
by large variations in hearing and patients will occasionally
present with a sudden deterioration. However, most will
also fluctuate naturally back to their original levels.

Drugs, especially the small group of ototoxic (ear-
damaging) antibiotics, may be a cause. Fortunately, however, this serious side effect is well known and such drugs are
used only in strictly necessary cases. A great deal of care is
taken to control the blood levels of the antibiotic and keep it
below the known toxic dose.

Rupture of the round or oval window may occasionally occur and is referred to as a *fistula*. This simply means that perilymph (the fluid surrounding the delicate inner ear membranes within the bony cochlea) manages to find its way from the inner ear into the middle ear via a rupture of either the oval or the round window (see Fig. 1). If this happens then a sudden, often severe sensorineural loss occurs and occasionally dizziness is a feature. How these fistulae occur is not quite clear, but quite often there is a preceding history of physical exertion or sudden change of pressure. Straining, as might happen when lifting heavy objects, pulling up roots, during childbirth, or even with severe coughing and sneezing has been implicated. Sudden pressure changes may occur with underwater diving or sudden descent in an aircraft. Whatever the theories, it is an important diagnosis and needs to be considered in all who have a sudden sensorineural deafness following exertion, straining, or pressure changes.

TREATMENT

If a fistula is suspected, then it can only be confirmed surgically. This entails lifting up the ear-drum to inspect the membranes and sealing any leak, usually with a piece of fat. About 25 per cent of these cases recover after surgery. However, the most important factor in management prior to surgery is total bed rest and absolute peace and quiet. This may help natural healing of fistulae and progress can be monitored with regular hearing tests. If a fistula is a possibility it is reasonable to wait a week after the onset of the deafness with the patient completely rested before deciding that spontaneous recovery is not taking place, in which case surgery is justified. Bed rest is also an important part of the management of other causes of sudden sensorineural deafness mentioned earlier.

Apart from fistulae of the round or oval windows, most

cases will have no obvious explanation as to their cause and treatment is often designed to include all known causes, in an attempt to cover all possibilities. This may sound confusing but it is the best that can be offered at present, and since many will recover with the treatment suggested, it is well worth trying. Treatment includes the use of steroid drugs if the cause is thought to be due to a virus affecting the auditory nerve, and they seem to be useful. The dose is large and is reduced over ten days. Blood vessel treatments are designed to open up the walls of the arteries to improve blood flow. This can be carried out by the use of vasodilator drugs, the most powerful of which is carbon dioxide. This is delivered as a 10 per cent mixture with air from a cylinder via a face mask for ten minutes every hour. Headaches and flushing of the face are occasional side effects. To improve the flow of blood, to reduce the stickiness of the red cells, and allow better perfusion of the inner ear, intravenous treatment with high molecular weight dextran can be tried.

All these treatments are largely based on educated guesswork and are best administered in hospital with serial daily hearing tests to assess progress. If some recovery has not begun to occur in ten days, then it is unlikely to do so and, apart from those with fistulae of their round or oval window membranes in whom operation is considered, there is no other treatment.

The hearing loss is often too severe for hearing aids but is nearly always only one sided. If both ears are affected, urgent rehabilitation of the unfortunate patient is required.

15

NOISE

Noise probably has a greater physical effect on people than does any other pollutant in the modern environment. Since the industrial revolution the harmful effects of noise on the ear have been publicized, yet most people are still blissfully unaware of the long term damage being done to hearing by everyday exposure from factories, engines, gunfire, discotheques, etc. Noise-induced deafness, like *presbycusis* (ageing deafness), cannot be cured; unlike the latter, however, it can be prevented.

INCIDENCE

The exact number of those suffering from noise-induced deafness is not known. This is because it is very difficult to distinguish between natural ageing and earlier exposure to noise; however, if noise exposure has been a prominent feature in early life then the natural ageing process often occurs at a younger age. The number of compensation claims throughout the world is increasing. In the USA, war pensions resulting from the Vietnam war are dominated by those claiming noise-induced deafness. In the UK about 10 000 people suffer from noise-induced deafness, and in the USA, in 1973, over 14 million workers were exposed daily to noise levels above the safety margin. In Canada 2500 new claims for compensation were filed in the province of Ontario alone in 1976.

HISTORICAL ASPECTS

The Bronze Age, with the discovery of metals and their subsequent hammering and shaping into weapons and tools, was probably the start of noise pollution. Biblical references to noise are found with reference to trumpets shattering the walls of Jericho and the horn of Alexander the Great calling to soldiers ten miles away. The book of Ecclesiasticus describes 'the smith sitting by the anvil, the noise of the hammer and anvil is ever in his ears—without these cannot a city be inhabited'. Pliny the elder in the first century AD in his 'natural history' noted deafness amongst those living near waterfalls on the Nile. Ear protection was recommended for those workers who hammered copper for a living as long ago as 1713. Blacksmiths' deafness has also long been recognized.

The industrial revolution heralded widespread noise pollution. 'Boiler-makers' deafness' became a well-used term at this time to describe the deafness induced by riveting, which was endemic in heavy engineering and ship-building areas of the UK such as Glasgow. In 1882, hearing loss from gun-fire was reported by Admiral Lord Rodney who was deafened for 14 days after firing 80 broadsides from his ship HMS Formidable.

HOW DOES NOISE CAUSE DEAFNESS?

A sudden blast of noise can occasionally rupture the ear-drum, but most loud and continuous industrial and environmental noise is transmitted via the ear-drum and middle ear ossicles directly to the cochlea (inner ear). In particular it strikes the part of the inner ear membrane responsible for high frequency hearing. This damages the hair cells responsible for higher frequency hearing (4 kHz) and an early sign is a dip on hearing testing, as seen in Fig. 20. It is interesting

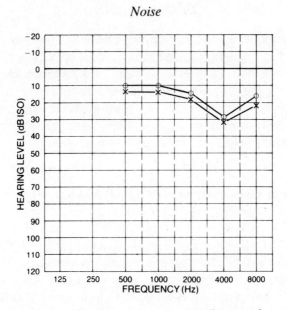

Fig. 20 Typical 4kHz dip on pure-tone audiogram due to noise.

but strange to note that some workers in heavy industry have 'resistant ears' and show very little sign of hearing loss compared with others in the same conditions, indicating that they have some inbuilt protection.

A natural protective reflex exists to give some protection against loud sound in normal ears when noise over 80 dB is heard. In response to this volume of noise a small muscle attached to the stapes contracts, preventing movement of the stapes. This cuts down some of the onward transmission of sound. Although this is a protective reflex, it tires very easily and when presented with continuous sound ceases to be effective.

Another important feature in whether a person suffers noise damage or not seems to be the gaps of quietness in between the noise. For instance, a rock musician on a stage for three hours with a 21-hour gap may be much less affected than a factory worker in less intense, but continuous, noise for eight hours with only a 16-hour rest.

It is probable (see Chapter 17 on ageing ears) that noise

damage increases the age-induced hearing loss if an elderly person has been exposed to noise as part of his working life, and in compensation claims these two factors have to be balanced. Fig. 21 shows the onward progression of noise damage if workers are not properly protected; the final result shows a more severe deafness than can be expected from natural ageing of the ears alone.

WHAT ARE THE SIGNS OF DAMAGING NOISE LEVELS?

Most of us will have had experience of a sudden loud noise causing us to feel a bit deaf immediately afterwards, occasionally with some ringing in the ears (tinnitus). Our hearing normally recovers, but if we were to have had an audiogram during this period it would have shown slight dullness of the hearing in the high frequencies. This is known as a '*tempor-*

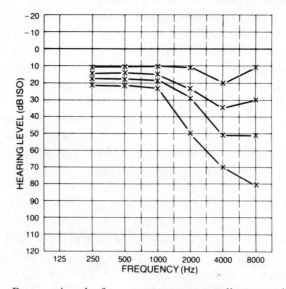

Fig. 21 Progressive deafness on pure-tone audiogram with years of exposure to dangerous noise.

ary threshold shift' and indicates we have been exposed to harmful noise. In sudden, loud explosions, for instance, there may well be a very long period of temporary threshold shift and recovery may not take place for a number of days. Prolonged periods of temporary threshold shift can also be seen at the end of a particularly noisy eight-hour factory shift. The workers all appear to shout at each other, and at their spouses when they get home for an hour or two afterwards. This is because they temporarily cannot hear so well and are unable to monitor the loudness of their own voice. They hear their own voice as being quiet and so raise it to what they think is normal, but others perceive it as being too loud. Eventually this temporary threshold shift may become permanent; it is then called noise-induced deafness. This is one of the problems of regulating factory noise, since if a temporary threshold shift always resulted in a permanent hearing loss this finding alone would be enough to reduce compulsorily the noise levels in factories, or remove those workers from that part of the factory. This does not necessarily always happen, however, since different people have different susceptibilities to the harmful effects of the same sound level.

It is a good rule that if you are suffering temporary threshold shift, even though others are not, it is likely that that particular noise is causing *you* harm.

THE EFFECTS OF NOISE-INDUCED DEAFNESS

The damage caused to the ear is an inner ear deafness. It is usually equal in both ears, except when it is caused by firearm shooting. Initially very little is noticed, but progressive loss of hearing occurs mainly in the high frequencies, giving rise to difficulty in hearing in groups of people speaking together. The symptoms are in fact similar to those of the ageing ear, except that they happen much earlier in life. Distressing tinnitus occasionally occurs. There is no cure and the answer is to prevent damage in the first place. Once deafness is established hearing aids are the only hope for help.

HOW MUCH NOISE IS SAFE?

There is a huge difference between steady state, low frequency noise in a factory, explosive noise, and pulsed noise as generated by pop groups. How much of each can be tolerated without damage is difficult to assess.

Factory noise

As a baseline, factory noise is worked out on a formula which allows a certain length of exposure to 90 dB in a 40-hour working week. It is a complicated formula and varies from industry to industry but is controlled by international standards.

Environmental noise

A new term has been developed to cover non-occupational noise—*sociocusis*. This includes everyday noise from cars, power tools, washing machines, etc., as well as those derived from music and sports.

Probably the biggest increase in urban noise levels has come from road transport. Although trucks consist of only about 20 per cent of the traffic, they produce 70 per cent of the noise. It is estimated that average noise levels outside the windows of a house on the side of a main road may reach 80 dB and underground railway networks very often exceed the 90 dB level. With respect to vehicles, there is often a feeling that silencing powerful machines reduces their performance; however, this has not been the case in aircraft design. The race-going public, on the one hand, has come to expect noisy racing motorcycles, and perhaps some of the excitement would be lost with quiet machines. The house-wife, however, might well choose to buy the quietest washing machine. Therefore our acceptance of noise levels from machines is a matter of both what we have come to expect from a particular machine and the job it does.

Power tools for the do-it-yourself enthusiast can be harm-ful, especially if used in confined spaces. It has been pointed out that many people who work in noise levels just below the dangerous limit for an eight-hour day often to come home and use a power tool for an hour or two at levels that put their total 24-hour exposure well into the danger zone.

Music does not seem to be enjoyable to some people unless it is played at full volume—perhaps it brings out some deep, rhythmic urge! There is an obvious difference between unamplified and amplified music. Whereas the noise level of an unamplified solo instrument player in a huge auditorium is acceptable, some pop music may be played in small rooms through very powerful amplifiers. Is the latter dangerous to hearing? It all depends on the length of exposure to danger-ous noise levels; it is therefore more likely to be a problem for the musician and 'disco' operator than the general pub-lic. It is possible that some pop groups can generate enough noise in a one-hour session to cause temporary threshold shift in the players and if this is not fully recovered before the next exposure then a definite risk is present. There are plenty of reported cases of noise-deafened performers. A study of students who frequently attended very loud pop concerts also showed a significant number with decreased hearing.

Interest has recently centred on the widespread use of personal stereo headphone cassette radios. In these the volume setting is often increased to overcome environ-mental noise. Of 190 college students in New York, 31 per cent exceeded the maximum allowable dose of noise and half of these exceeded the level by over 100 per cent. A smaller study in which volunteers were allowed to listen to their headsets for three hours at their usual maximum level indicated that a third of these showed temporary threshold shifts. It has been suggested that such radios should carry a health warning on purchase!

There is considerable world-wide effort being made to reduce sociocusis and this should make life not only quieter, but also less stressful.

Gunfire

In rural areas of the UK, shotgun shooting is responsible for a considerable amount of high frequency hearing loss in those who enjoy the sport. Recently there has been much more awareness of the harm it can do to hearing and ear defenders are at least being seen as acceptable on shoots. Often such people are also commonly exposed to farm machinery noise. Although tractor cabs are now quite well silenced, the damage is cumulative. Whereas most noise-induced hearing loss is symmetrical in both ears, the gun is normally held diagonal to the body. The ear nearest the butt of the gun on the shoulder is thus less likely to be damaged than the opposite one which is nearer the muzzle.

Military guns can generate enormous sudden sound levels, occasionally in the region of 180 dB. Twenty per cent of field gunners in the last war suffered permanent noise deafness after firing their first round. Military personnel are not only exposed to gunfire, but also to tanks and helicopters, which can be exceptionally noisy. However, there is an obvious difficulty in hearing military commands with ear protection in place.

PREVENTION AND PROTECTION

Sometimes excessive noise levels are unavoidable, in which case the ears must be protected. More often, however, the absolute levels can be reduced by better engineering design.

Reduction in noise

The first task in noise reduction is to measure the sound levels in industrial premises. This is a complex procedure since the levels are likely to vary. Some noises are continuous and others are intermittent; also workers will move from one position to another. It is useless to take a series of individual readings; the environment as a whole needs to be monitored for a full working day, followed by analysis done from tape recordings. Ideally, the results would show the length of time any employee could be expected to work safely at any position in the factory. However, a complicating issue, as mentioned before, is the variation in individual's susceptibility to noise damage. It is more practical to identify certain areas and pieces of machinery as carrying a risk. These can then be silenced, perhaps by enclosing them with soundproofing or by moving all the noisy machines to one area and operating them by remote control from a sound-proofed area. New equipment may need design modifications. Often simple things can be done; for instance, a diesel engine in a bus, or a boat mounted on steel frames, could have rubber mountings to separate the engine from its steel bed.

Testing of hearing

Widespread, simple audiometry can be done rapidly and needs to be repeated regularly, especially when workers change from one noisy job to another. It is not necessary to be too accurate, but merely to detect deterioration and to act when it occurs. Deterioration may mean that the employee is being damaged by noise or is refusing to wear the ear protection offered, in which case be needs advice otherwise he could not expect to be successful in a later compensation claim.

Protection

Apart from silencing machinery, the only other available

form of protection is personal protection with ear-plugs or ear-phones. There are many different devices available, but the greatest hurdle is to have them accepted as sensible, by the work-force. This requires careful explanation of the damage that can occur without them and management must be seen to set an example by using them too. Excuses are often heard, for example that the wearing of ear protection prevents them hearing shouted warnings of dangers, and many have considered that wearing ear protection is rather 'sissy'. In the UK the hunting and shooting fraternity have been as slow to accept hard hats for riding as they have ear protection for shooting, and repeated education is required.

Protection devices basically consist of ear-plugs or ear-muffs. Cotton wool is useless and fibre-glass wool types, although a bit better, can occasionally irritate the skin. Waxed wool is also available. Bungs to go in the ear are of two types: the first is made from foam which is compressed, inserted, and allowed to expand; the second is made from soft plastic or rubber, which is usually conical to allow easier fitting. They must be snugly fitting and can be uncomfortable at first. A small hole in the centre of the bung can let low frequency sound through so that the workers can hear commands and yet not be damaged by loud sounds. This type has been used in the armed forces.

Ear-muffs are the most effective type of protection. Complaints are that they are heavy, hot to wear, or difficult to use with spectacles. The pad is most effective if filled with fluid to allow a good seal around the ear. Sophisticated military muffs have a communication link built into them and are incorporated as part of a helmet.

No protection is perfect. The best muffs can cut out only 50 dB in the high frequencies, and considerably less reduction is obtainable from ear-plugs. Inefficient use, either because of poor placement of the plugs or because of the muffs not being sealed when worn with glasses or over long hair, considerably reduces their effectiveness—it is no good just issuing protection without explanation as to its correct use. Reducing the sound at source is the best answer. Finally, it is often assumed that because someone already has a hearing loss he will not hear noise so loudly and therefore will not be damaged: this is nonsense.

16

TINNITUS

Tinnitus is not a disease, but is a most wretched symptom for which the sufferer deserves every sympathy. It is the term used for noises heard in the head or ear. Except in very rare cases, it is only the victim who can hear the noise. Tinnitus can be extremely bizarre, as has been shown by people who have reproduced their tinnitus using music synthesizers. The intensity of the sound can also be severe, certainly loud enough to interfere with day-to-day life, and may be constantly present.

We probably all have tinnitus from time to time. The thumping in our ears after exercise could be classed as tinnitus. However, we must remember that the bone of the skull housing the ear is surrounded by very large blood vessels going to the brain, so it is hardly surprising we occasionally hear the noise of the blood passing through these vessels, particularly when blood-pressure is raised from exercise. Intractable tinnitus is a completely different matter. It can sometimes come from problems associated with the blood vessels, but in most cases its origin is in the hearing mechanism itself.

WHERE DOES TINNITUS ORIGINATE?

We are still unable to say with certainty where most cases of tinnitus originate, although the vast majority are thought to be caused by damage to some of the tiny hair cells of the cochlea. However, even in known cases of cochlea damage this is not the whole answer. Some unfortunate patients may plead to have their ear destroyed or the auditory nerve cut in the hope of relieving the tinnitus. This would seem perfectly logical, for if the tinnitus originated from the inner ear then destruction of the latter should relieve it, but this is not the case. Many investigators feel there must be some brain pathway involved that is not completely understood. Recent important research using powerful microphones and amplifiers placed in the external ear-canal has picked up noise generated by the cochlea in patients with tinnitus. These are referred to as *cochlear echoes* and this will hopefully lead to a better understanding and more efficient treatment of this distressing symptom.

CAUSES OF TINNITUS

The external and middle ear may have problems of which tinnitus is one of the symptoms. Simple causes such as wax, middle ear fluid (glue ear), otosclerosis, and chronic infection in the middle ear are examples and all are, of course, remedial to treatment.

Tinnitus arising from the inner ear is not easy to cure, but in most cases can be helped.

Noise

Damage to the inner ear through noise is very frequently associated with tinnitus, although the latter symptom may come many years after the original damage has occurred and be most distressing to the sufferer in later life. Better public awareness of noise and the damaging effects it can have on the ear is emphasized in Chapter 15; it is sufficient to say here that the symptom of tinnitus has been largely underestimated by those working in noisy environments. Even in industrial compensation cases brought by people who have had their hearing damaged by noise, little importance is placed on the symptom of tinnitus. Noise damage disrupts the tiny hair cells of the cochlea at its high frequency end and often a high-pitched tinnitus results. It is essential that proper ear-defenders are used for shooting and working with noisy machinery. Full volume on personal cassette radios played through ear-phones should be avoided, and special care also needs to be taken by rock musicians and those running discotheques if tinnitus is not to be a problem in later life.

Drugs

It is well recognized that certain drugs may cause tinnitus. The best example is aspirin given in large doses to patients suffering from rheumatoid arthritis. This type of tinnitus is usually reversible and patients can often control the dose so that they stay below the level which causes it. The other classical tinnitus-causing drug is quinine, which is often used in the prevention of malaria. Some antibiotics which can damage the inner ear (ototoxic) produce deafness and dizziness, and also tinnitus, as the main symptoms.

Menière's disease

This disease has been referred to in detail in Chapter 13. It produces a characteristic, usually low frequency tinnitus which fluctuates. Patients will often describe the tinnitus as becoming much louder immediately prior to an attack of severe dizziness, and this is usually also accompanied by a diminution of hearing. It is very difficult to predict what will happen to the tinnitus in Menière's disease patients, but many will recover. However, even in those who are offered surgical treatment for their Menière's disease, there can be no absolute certainty that the tinnitus will be helped. Because the tinnitus gets worse during an attack, abolition of the attacks allows the tinnitus to be coped with more easily.

Other diseases

In the absence of any obvious cause relating to the ears, generalized disease such as anaemia, raised blood-pressure, and an underfunctioning thyroid gland should be excluded as a cause for tinnitus. It is a misconception amongst the lay public that brain tumours present with tinnitus. This happens extremely rarely, but is something that is at the back of most patients minds and this fear needs to be allayed at the beginning of a consultation.

HEARING AND TINNITUS

Some people seem to have absolutely normal hearing and yet have quite severe tinnitus; these are a particularly dif-ficult group of sufferers to account for. Only a small proportion of such patients eventually go on to have a hearing loss.

The majority of those with tinnitus have, of course, some hearing loss and the causes have been mentioned. Most will also say that as their hearing loss increases, perhaps with natural ageing, the tinnitus appears to get a bit worse. Some of the severest cases are seen in patients with no hearing at all in the affected ear.

WHAT CAN BE DONE TO HELP?

The tinnitus sufferer is very understandably distressed and sometimes depressed by this symptom; sympathetic understanding of the problem is essential. Reassurance that there is no serious underlying disease may be all that is required to allay the fears of the patient and help him cope with the symptoms. An example of the wrong approach is to say 'You have tinnitus and must learn to live with it'.

A proper examination of the ear and hearing function will elicit those causes mentioned earlier which can be readily treated. It will also give the clinician a much better idea of the help that could be offered to the patient.

Hearing aids and tinnitus maskers

Since many cases of tinnitus become worse as hearing loss increases, for instance with age, then it would seem reasonable to boost the hearing level by the use of a hearing aid. Indeed, simply allowing more sound to come into the ear will effectively mask the tinnitus in a large number of patients and have the added benefit of improving the hearing as well.

Tinnitus maskers look very like behind-the-ear hearing aids; they are basically noise generators which feed a rushing sound into the ear to mask the tinnitus. The process by which this works is not fully understood, especially as low levels of a broad-band rushing noise can effectively mask a high-pitched tinnitus of a completely different frequency. It is important that these instruments are not used with a tight-fitting hearing aid mould, which would otherwise reduce hearing. Usually the masking sound enters the ear with an open tube or mould. Recently tinnitus maskers have been developed to generate different masking tones in the hope of matching them to the tinnitus tone heard by the patient. The fitting of a tinnitus masker has to be accompanied by very careful follow-up if the patient is to accept it as a useful instrument. It is no good expecting the patient to walk into a hearing aid dealer, collect a masker, and have it work without guidance—thorough back-up is essential. Many patients find that by wearing the masker for 2 or 3 hours the tinnitus is completely or partially suppressed for a period of time even after the masker is removed. The duration of relief varies very much from patient to patient. Some are never completely relieved but do prefer the masking noise to their own tinnitus. Many tinnitus sufferers will find that they can cope perfectly well during their day-to-day life because of masking from background environmental noise, but will be irritated by their tinnitus while trying to go to sleep or when it is quiet and will wear their masking devices at those times. There are also so-called 'pillow maskers'; these fit underneath the patient's pillow, generating masking noise which will help blot out the tinnitus when trying to go to sleep. Some people find that just simply keeping a loudly ticking clock in the bedroom or even a clock radio, which will switch itself off when they are asleep, is quite sufficient as a masking device to help at night.

Drug treatment

There has been a lot of interest recently in drug therapy. Unfortunately, however, the only drug which seems to be effective lasts for a very short time and has to be given via an intravenous route. This is a local anaesthetic drug called lignocaine. Related drugs can be obtained in pill form but are disappointingly ineffective. Tranquillizers serve only to diminish the importance of the tinnitus in the patient's mind and do not treat the condition itself. At present there is no effective drug therapy for tinnitus.

Other treatments

Dietary changes have been reported to be useful by some patients. This mainly consists of reducing the levels of caffeine in coffee and sometimes avoiding dairy products. Smoking does not help because it tends to narrow the blood vessels, reducing the blood supply to the inner ear. Alcohol in moderation dilates blood vessels and possibly improves tinnitus, but care must be taken not to end up as an alcoholic!

Stress certainly seems to make tinnitus worse. If it is possible to change the tinnitus sufferer's lifestyle to reduce the amount of stress this can often be an important factor. Many people will find relief from relaxation or yoga classes.

Alternative medicine may be used, including homoeopathic extract of ginkgo (maidenhair tree), but its effectiveness has not been proved. Acupuncture is also reported to work in some instances. Since these treatments do no harm, they may well be worth exploring.

WHAT OF THE FUTURE?

The quest for a drug which will help tinitus will undoubtedly continue. Maskers are being improved all the time and the ability for the patient to adjust the masking tone to suit their tinnitus is being explored at the moment.

Electrical stimulation by small electrodes inserted into the cochlea can abolish tinnitus, but at the moment is only suitable for those patients who have a total absence of hearing since electrode insertion necessarily destroys any remaining hearing. Electrical stimulation of the cochlea with electrodes placed over the skin behind the ear is being investigated and may offer some hope.

Self-help groups

The UK patient self-help group is the British Tinnitus Association. It was founded by Jack Ashley, MP, in 1979. There are about 80 branches and a regular news-letter is published which gives up-to-date information on developments for patients. The address is given in the appendix.

To summarize, tinnitus is a common and distressing symptom. However, about 60 per cent of cases can be helped by proper management.

17

AGEING EARS

Few of us, if we live long enough, will escape the effect of ageing on our ears. This is called *presbycusis* (from the Greek *presbus* meaning 'old man' and *cusis* meaning 'hearing') and is a perfectly natural process (Fig. 22). Just as all our body tissues gradually degenerate with age, so the ear is no exception. However, the degree of hearing loss varies considerably from person to person. It is estimated that seven out of ten people over the age of 70 are handicapped by poor hearing. In our constantly ageing society this is becoming a major medical problem and one which deserves much more attention than is at present paid to it.

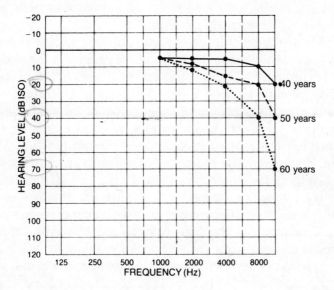

Fig. 22 Audiogram showing normal deterioration with ageing.

If all body tissues deteriorate with age, then it is difficult
to understand why some elderly people retain excellent
hearing into very old age while others have a severe handicap. It is also difficult to know at what age normal deterioration in hearing begins, but the overall trend is for the high
tones to be heard gradually less well than the low. One of
the problems with large, so-called 'normal' studies is to
know whether they are truly representative of simple ageing
or whether there are other factors that might be increasing
the hearing loss. Such factors might include genetic influences, diet, and most importantly environmental noise. It
is well recognized that men fare worse than women with
regard to high frequency hearing loss. It is usually assumed
that men have been involved in noisy occupations, but there
is little knowledge of the effect of everyday noise such as
washing machines, cars, and loud music. Tests among rural
tribes who have not been subjected to environmental noise
show that they have much better hearing than urban dwel-
lers, with women and men having equally good hearing. It is
therefore probable that noise is a major factor in increasing
the severity of normal age-related deafness.

Although the middle ear structures also age, the ear-drum
losing its elasticity and the joints of the ossicles in the middle
ear becoming a bit stiffer, this causes relatively little loss of
hearing compared with inner ear changes. Unfortunately,
wear and tear in the inner ear means loss of the vital cells on
the organ of Corti which cannot reproduce themselves.
Hence there is a progressive deterioration in function. It is
generally agreed that there are four distinct types of change
occurring in the inner ear. They are said to give differing
hearing patterns ranging from a fairly flat loss across all
frequencies to good hearing in the low frequencies but a very
severe deafness in the high frequencies. Not only are the
pure-tone audiograms variable, but the ability to discrimin-
ate speech varies enormously between one person and
another and seems to bear little relation to the shape of the
audiogram. One would assume that a flat type of hearing

loss across all frequencies would be easy to correct with a hearing aid and that a sharply sloping curve would not, but this is not necessarily the case. Very often even those with the most disastrous-looking hearing tests can be helped considerably by a hearing aid.

SYMPTOMS

Difficulty in discriminating speech leads, unfortunately, to frustration and a muddled embarrassment for the elderly person with a hearing loss. This frequently results in a real fear of making inappropriate comments, leading to that person withdrawing from conversation and becoming isolated from society. It is very often the family that asks for help rather than the patient. Although many elderly people will appear to be hearing perfectly normally in a one-to-one situation in a quiet room, they are often hopelessly lost in a crowd where there are many people talking at once—so-called 'cocktail-party deafness'. Many sufferers also say that children's and female voices are less easy to hear than men's, as are telephone bells and bird-song. All these symptoms are suggestive of a high frequency hearing loss. We are all familiar with the elderly person cupping his ear in the hope of directing more sound into it and this may have the beneficial effect of making the speaker talk more slowly and clearly. However, if speaker raises his voice the response is often 'don't shout, I'm not deaf'. This is because of a phenomenon called *recruitment*, in which if the voice is raised too much it is heard not as clear words, but a painful cacophony of undifferentiated sound. This phenomenon also makes the fitting and adjustment of hearing aids difficult. However, as will be seen in Chapter 18, there are many different types of aids with differing amounts of frequency selection, and with patience it is usually possible to find an instrument that is of great benefit to the elderly person. Before hearing aids can be accepted, however, the stigma of becoming deaf has to be

overcome by society. Only when there is greater understanding of the elderly person's problems will the above
symptoms become less of a burden to the patient.

DIAGNOSIS

The diagnosis of presbycusis is one of exclusion. It is strongly
recommended that all elderly people who feel they have a
hearing loss are examined carefully by an ear specialist, who
will not only take a full history, but also examine the ears
and carry out at least pure-tone hearing testing. Very occasionally other causes of hearing loss are encountered which
need much fuller investigation and treatment other than the
supply of a hearing aid.

WHAT CAN BE DONE?

If you are an elderly person reading this chapter, then you
should realize that hearing deterioration can almost be
regarded as normal and that you are one of millions with
similar difficulties. Better public awareness will hopefully be
your greatest ally, not necessarily for the sympathy but
simply the recognition of your handicap so that you are
given time and understanding. The symbol of the 'sympathetic hearing scheme' is:

You will often see these signs displayed in shops, banks, and offices and it means that the staff employed are willing to make your life easier by taking a little more trouble. If this type of scheme spreads then your life should be easier.

You should also realize that you may be making life a little more difficult for your family if they have to keep repeating themselves, and upsetting for you if you keep getting the 'wrong end of the stick'. Therefore you should allow yourself to be assessed with hearing tests and for consideration of treatment. Unfortunately, there is no scientific evidence that any medical treatment is effective. Patients are frequently advised to try various vitamins and herbal remedies. Although no harm will come of taking these under proper supervision, it is wrong to expect miraculous cures. The same holds true for acupuncture and any form of surgery. While the medical and the paramedical services are unable to carry out any restoration of hearing, there are a tremendous number of aids and services that can make the life of a hearing-impaired person more tolerable.

Hearing aids are discussed fully in Chapter 18. As will be seen, they range enormously in type. It is hoped that, after examination by a clinician and appropriate hearing tests, the correct type of hearing aid can be fitted first time around, but this is by no means always the case. The most important advice for the new hearing aid wearer is to be persistent. It takes time to get used to a hearing aid. However, with help from professionals and, if necessary, repeated switching of different types of aid until one is found that is suitable, most patients find a hearing aid to be of enormous benefit. Other important gadgets (which are also discussed in the hearing aid chapter) may well include door or telephone bells of different tones and special television aerials to make reception better.

Apart from hearing aids, a good deal of help can be obtained from learning basic lip-reading skills. The local hearing-aid supplier, whether in a hospital or commercial premises, should be able to supply names of local lip-reading teachers. Much of the time, the understanding of speech is derived not only from what we hear, but also from the expression on the face and the movement of the lips. It is therefore important to make sure that the hearing aid wearer can adequately see the speaker. In noisy surroundings hearing aids will tend to pick up background sound and can be irritating. With practice, however, this can be overcome to a large extent. It is also important not to be sitting or standing in the corner of the room where sound can easily be reflected off the walls. More advice of this type will be found in Chapter 18.

Above all it is hoped that the elderly person will seek and accept help to avoid withdrawal from society and that one day hearing aids will be as acceptable as false teeth and spectacles.

18

AIDS TO HEARING

The provision of a standard hearing aid is only a small part
of the total range of services available to the hard of hearing.
Yet all too often a hearing aid is supplied and the patient
is given very little guidance. This is tragic, because little
benefit will be gained and the aid will most probably end up
in the dressing table drawer.

HEARING AIDS

Hearing aids are amplification systems designed to improve
the auditory signals experienced in everyday life. They cannot restore normal hearing, but do allow most people with a
hearing impairment to overcome the worst effects of their
hearing loss. There are so many different models of aid
available that only a brief description of the different cate-
gories is possible here. In the UK there is a dilemma
between choosing from one of the NHS instruments or in-
vesting, often heavily, in a commercial aid.

The advantage of a NHS aid is that it is supplied free to
the patient, as are future servicing and supply of batteries.
There are now some 13 different models available with different specifications to suit different hearing losses. Most
people will benefit from a small behind-the-ear aid, which
looks almost identical to any commercial aid. The only type
of aid not supplied, unless there are good medical indications, is the 'in-the-ear' aid, which is certainly cosmetic but
may not be adequate in power output for more than moderate losses. The other major advantage of the NHS aid is that

if one model is not suitable then different types can be tried until the patient is satisfied with no cost to them. However, reputable dealers in the commercial field will always operate some form of free trial period. This is essential, for although there are now machines available to help decide which hearing aid is best for particular types of hearing loss, the best test is wearer satisfaction. This is probably best done by the wearer using the hearing aid in his own environment, be it a work-place, home, theatre, etc., before deciding. This is because there will be a difference in performance in these situations compared with an acoustically deadened hearing aid dealer's premises. There is a wide range of excellent quality commercial aids available and, as mentioned before, it is the only way at present in the UK of obtaining in-the-ear aids. Although most dealers are excellent and totally reliable, as in any profession there are a few rogues, and the advice of your doctor or personal recommendation from friends is probably the best way of choosing, rather than answering newspaper advertisements. Before a hearing aid can be supplied, an accurate hearing test in a sound-proof booth should be performed so that the provision of the aid can be matched to the loss. This always happens in the NHS, but may not occur in all commercial establishments. The major disadvantage of the NHS aid is the occasional lengthy delay in hearing aid provision.

TYPES OF HEARING AID

Mechanical

Very rarely there are indications to supply old-fashioned ear-trumpets. They provide some amplification without any electrical distortion. For those with very arthritic hands, for instance, they are less fiddly to use.

Electrical

With improvements in the field of microelectronics, hearing

aids have become more miniature and sophisticated. All hearing aids basically consist of a microphone to pick up sound, an amplifier to make it louder, and an ear-phone to feed the sound into the ear. They use batteries as a power source and, whether body worn, behind, or in the ear, they all need these basic components.

Body worn

Body-worn hearing aids (Plate X) are much less commonly prescribed nowadays since miniaturization has made possible the more cosmetically acceptable behind- and in-the-ear aids. Apart from this cosmetic disadvantage, body-worn aids also suffer from the microphone being worn on the chest and often hidden by clothes. This may occlude the microphone from incoming sound and may also pick up unwanted rustling from clothes rubbing.

However, for the profoundly deaf, much greater power can be obtained from these instruments and the long separation of the ear-piece from the microphone minimizes the whistling sound generated by feedback that can occur with ear-level instruments. Secondly, the large controls make it easier to handle by those with stiff hands or poor vision.

Bone conducting

In some unfortunate people who have chronically discharging ears or congenital or traumatic absence of the external ear and ear-canal, an aid applied to the bone behind the ear will conduct sound to the inner ear. Usually, these are fitted as a tight headband attached to a body-worn aid (Plate XI). More recently hearing aids that screw directly into the skull have been designed and are an extremely efficient way of overcoming this problem (see Chapter 19). Another way of using a bone-conducting aid is to incorporate it into a heavy spectacle frame, the arm of the spectacles applying pressure contact to the bone.

Behind the ear

This type of aid is by far the most commonly prescribed aid (Plate XII). It is cosmetically acceptable, there is no connecting cord, and the microphone is at a more logical place (i.e. the ear). With well-fitting moulds, acoustic feedback (whistling) is minimized, even if powerful aids are necessary to correct the deafness. Possible disadvantages of these aids include the need for greater manipulative skills in placing the aid and adjusting the controls. Also, whereas body-worn aids use standard AA batteries, camera- or watch-type ('button') batteries are needed for the behind-the-ear aids and are less readily available. Many behind-the-ear aids are now extremely sophisticated and not only amplify selectively at frequencies lacking in the patient, but have volume, tone, and inductive loop controls (T-setting). This enables better hearing on the telephone, in public places, and when watching television, etc. (see below).

In-the-ear

These aids are becoming very popular because of their small size, their simple on/off control, and the ease of insertion (Plate XIII) The microphone, amplifier, and battery compartments are all housed in the mould; therefore, once made, fitting adjustments to the mould are very difficult. They are not yet routinely available on the NHS and are probably only suitable for moderate losses since the problem of acoustic feedback (whistling) arises where the microphone and amplifier are close together, which limits the power output of these aids.

Radio aids

These aids (Plate XIV) are particularly useful in the classroom. The system works as follows. The child may be fitted with a behind-the-ear aid which has a socket for direct input of radio transmissions into the amplifier. Usually the child also wears an FM radio receiver on his chest, with a lead directly connected to the socket in the hearing aid amplifier behind his ear. The teacher wears a radio microphone FM transmitter which broadcasts to the child's radio receiver. The great advantage of this system is that the teacher's instructions are transmitted directly to the child's ear at a considerable range without the child picking up unwanted background sound.

EAR-MOULDS

The ear-mould is a moulded plastic ear-piece; it is a very important part of the hearing aid system. It is through a small hollow channel in the mould that the sound from the aid is delivered to the ear. Every ear is a different shape so the mould has to be tailor made. A snug fit is vital if acoustic feedback (whistling) is to be avoided when the volume is turned up. The first stage in fitting the hearing aid is to make the mould. The technician will inject soft, semiliquid silicone mixed with a curing agent into the ear-canal and inside of the pinna. After a short while this sets and then can easily be removed. This is an accurate cast of the outer ear and canal. The cast is then sent away to be manufactured into the final mould, which is usually made out of acrylic, but other softer materials are sometimes indicated. Not only is it important that the mould fits correctly, but it must also be kept clean. Regular washing in soapy water is all that is required, having first detached the electronics! The central sound channel must be kept clear of wax, and pipe cleaners are useful for this purpose.

BATTERIES

Body-worn aids use AA type batteries; these are widely available and long-life ones are probably best. However, they suddenly lose their power when exhausted, so spares should always be carried. Old batteries must be removed from the aid in case they should leak.

Behind-the-ear aids use the button-type batteries found in cameras, calculators, and watches. There are a number of different types, the most powerful being silver oxide, but the zinc–air type has a longer life. Full advice will be given by the hearing-aid dealer. These batteries must be disposed of correctly as they contain harmful chemicals and it is best to keep the old ones in their container. In the NHS system old batteries must be returned to the hearing aid department before issue of new ones can be made. There have been reports of children swallowing batteries, which is obviously dangerous, and they must be kept out of reach of little hands.

Hearing aid fault check

Fault	Solution
Fading sound	Replace battery
No sound	(1) Check controls are on and volume is turned up
	(2) Is there a battery?
	(3) Is the battery the right way round?
	(4) Is the mould blocked with wax?
	(5) Is the tube connecting the aid to the mould kinked?
	(6) Is the tube full of condensation? If so, blow through it until this disappears
	(7) Replace the cord of body-worn aids

Other problems

Whistling

The mould is probably not fitting properly or the volume is turned up too high. A new mould may be required.

Clothes rub

Body-worn aids suffer from this problem; it may be necessary to resite the hearing aid box.

Irritation in the ears

Allergy to mould material occasionally occurs. Pain and discharge in the ear are most likely to be due to inflammation of the outer ear-canal (external otitis) and are often due to the ear not being able to 'breathe' because of the occluding mould. This allows it to become hot and sticky and gives rise to skin infection. Dirty moulds can be a precipitating factor. A doctor should be consulted if the condition occurs.

OTHER AIDS TO HEARING

Loop system

Most hearing aids have a 'T' (for Telecoil) setting on their controls. This activates a pick-up coil which can respond to changing magnetic fields. In the so-called 'loop system' a loop of wire is fixed around the inside of the periphery of public buildings—for example churches, classrooms, theatres, etc.—this loop can be connected to the amplifier of the microphone being used by a speaker in that building (e.g. a teacher, actor, etc.). The changing magnetic fields from the loop of wire can be received and converted back into sound by the induction coil in the hearing aid. The great advantage of this system is that background noise is reduced, the wearer being able to concentrate directly on the words spoken into the microphone.

Many *telephones* can be adapted to allow the 'T' setting to pick up sound more clearly.

A dealer can adapt a *television* to work off a loop aerial in much the same way.

Door bells

Changing the frequency of a door bell from a high to a low frequency may help those with a high frequency deafness. An alternative is to connect the bell ringing with lights flashing on and off. The same can apply to telephone bells.

Vibrating alarms

An alarm clock, for instance, can be connected to a vibrating pad. When the alarm goes off the vibrating pad placed in a suitable spot (e.g. under the pillow) alerts the hearing-impaired person.

Lip reading

Most of us use a primitive form of lip reading, or at least the reading of face patterns when speaking to each other in a noisy room. There is no doubt that the teaching of proper lip reading to those with an increasing hearing loss can be an enormous aid to hearing. In the UK, lip-reading classes are normally held at the local adult education centres; information on them can be found in the nearest NHS hearing aid clinic.

Sympathetic hearing scheme

The symbol of the sympathetic hearing scheme is as follows:

It is now being found in many shops, banks, public buildings, telephone boxes, etc., and it indicates that the hard of hearing are thoughtfully catered for. There may be a specific staff training or an induction loop fitted into the building. This scheme is especially useful in places such as banks and post offices where there are glass partitions and it is hoped that the system will continue to spread.

DO'S AND DON'TS FOR THOSE SPEAKING TO THE HEARING IMPAIRED

Do

1. Face the light so that you can be seen easily by the hearing-impaired person.

2. Speak clearly and naturally and look directly at the person.

3. Be friendly, casual, and tolerant.

4. Have sympathetic understanding, but not pity.

5. Be patient with mistakes.

6. Watch for signs of fatigue.

7. Write 'key words' on a pad. This is especially important with proper names.

8. Don't change the subject matter suddenly; make sure the subject is understood before engaging in long conversations.

Don't

1. Mumble.

2. Exaggerate your lip movements.

3. Put your hand over your mouth when talking.

4. Shout.

5. Have a cigarette in your mouth, or blow a smoke screen in front of your face.

6. Repeat the same word over and over again. Try changing the wording since some words are difficult to see on the lips.

7. Wear dark glasses; much can be said by your eyes.

Finally, the stigma of deafness must be overcome. As we all live longer, most of us will find difficulty with our hearing with advancing years. This must be accepted as being perfectly natural. The hard of hearing must not be afraid to say that they have a problem, as this makes it easier for everyone.

19

THE FUTURE

PREVENTION OF DEAFNESS

One of the successes of modern preventative medicine is the reduction in the incidence of children born with severe hearing loss. This is primarily a result of the prevention of rubella affecting mothers in the first three months of pregnancy. This has been achieved by widespread vaccination of non-immune teenage girls. In the UK this has had the effect of reducing the number of pupils who need special education because of hearing loss. Improved neonatal care, with the emergence of highly specialized intensive care units for the new-born and particularly those who are premature, has undoubtedly prevented many cases of deafness. This is the result of careful attention to the oxygen requirements, monitoring of potentially dangerous antibiotics, and conquering of neonatal jaundice.

Probably the biggest menace that still needs to be conquered is the damage done to the ears by noise. Widespread noise protection policies are in action in industry, but better public awareness is still needed to avoid hearing loss caused by 'social' noise.

SURGERY

Modern microsurgery for the middle ear has advanced to such a degree that little more at present can be done to improve the techniques, apart from the development of new materials for use as replacement ossicles. Various plastic and carbon fibre materials have been tried and, more recently, ceramics have been assessed. Unfortunately, on a global scale the vast majority of patients with hearing impairment do not have a deafness that is amenable to repair by surgery. In other words, it is not the middle ear which causes the vast majority of hearing loss, but the inner ear and auditory nerve. Research attention has been drawn to this large group to try to improve their lot. In general, this requires the improvement of hearing aids and the development of cochlear implants.

HEARING AIDS

With the rapid advance in the development of microelectronics, it sometimes seems that the hearing aid industry has been left behind. However, the problems in designing an instrument that will correct a hearing loss which is different in each individual patient are immense. One of the greatest problems that all hearing aid users mention is the unwanted ability of the hearing aid to pick up background noise. The idea of a 'thinking' hearing aid that can selectively distinguish between speech sounds and unwanted background noise needs to be developed in practice.

There are also those unfortunate patients who are unable to wear a hearing aid because of an associated external or middle ear problem, for instance, those born without ear-canals. The biggest group of people who could benefit from a hearing aid, but who are prevented from doing so, are those with chronically discharging middle ears through some middle ear or mastoid disease which, for some reason, is not amenable to medical or surgical treatment. Since in these circumstances hearing aid moulds become blocked by the discharge, the use of a bone-conducting hearing aid is one alternative. However, these hearing aids are uncomfortable to wear and contact with bone is not readily achievable because of the layer of skin and muscle between the loudspeaker of the hearing aid and the bone. A recent major advance has been the ability to attach the hearing aid directly into bone. This has been developed in Sweden and is known as a *bone-anchored hearing aid*. Its secret lies in the placement of a titanium device like a press-stud that is screwed into the bone and is not rejected by it. The patient then has the ability to clip the hearing aid directly on this titanium press-stud, which is visible as a small fitting behind the ear. The improved contact with bone gives a much better quality of sound reproduction. Similar magnetic devices are also being developed.

THE COCHLEAR IMPLANT

The subject of cochlear implantation is exciting and has generated a lot of press interest, but with some media articles have unfortunately raised false hopes in some patients. The subject must still be regarded as experimental; at present it is only of use in those totally deafened and then only as an aid to lip reading. It cannot usually restore the ability to hear speech. In those with even the smallest amount of residual hearing a powerful hearing aid is still the better answer. Considerable developments are taking place in the production of cochlear implants. At its present stage, however, the work is probably best left to those workers who have already developed some expertise in this field, in a few centres in the USA, Australia, the UK, and Europe. Most researchers agree that at the moment it is best to implant only those who have had hearing and speech prior to being rendered totally deaf, rather than those who have been born congenitally deaf and who have no previous knowledge of speech. Therefore the use of cochlear implants in children is still controversial.

What is a cochlear implant?

The object of a cochlear implant is to stimulate normal nerve fibres connecting the totally damaged cochlear to the brain by using electrodes placed in the cochlear. This is known as an *intracochlear implant*. However, since there are 32 000 nerve endings in the auditory nerve, the stimulation of all these fibres would need an impossibly complex multi-channel electrode. Even then it would not be possible to site it so as to line it up with all the appropriate nerve endings! The technique is invasive in that the cochlear has to be opened and occasional quite serious infective complications occur. Single or multi-channel electrodes have been used and, although multi-channel would seem to be more effective, the results are inconclusive. Another type of implant is the *extracochlear implant*. This is simply an electrode placed on the round window membrane. Although this needs a surgical operation to lift the ear-drum to site the electrode accurately, it does not puncture the round window as the intracochlear device does and is not inserted into the cochlea. This means that it is considerably safer and it is also easier to change. This last point is important because, in this rapidly developing field, better electrodes will become available and updating of implants in patients is desirable. It is difficult at the moment to prove that the results of this device are inferior to those with the intracochlear implant.

Who is able to benefit and what are the results from cochlear implantation?

Compared with the huge number of people with impaired hearing, only a very small proportion are suitable for implantation. Most teams inserting these devices have a rigorous screening procedure for selection. This includes extensive hearing testing, psychological assessment, and a very careful explanation of what to expect from the device. Usually only patients with total, bilateral deafness, but whose auditory nerve endings are functional, are suitable. They must also be prepared for extensive rehabilitation afterwards, with many hours of hard work with the researchers, to make the most effective use of the electrical signals.

Patients must understand that hearing of distinct speech is not going to be possible; however, awareness of environmental sounds such as traffic, doorbells, and even the ability to recognize familiar voices may be achieved. The technique may also be a useful aid to lip-reading and it seems to help some people to produce better intonation in their speech. Some patients also report a decrease in the level of tinnitus. World-wide there are some remarkable 'show' patients who seem to be able to obtain a great deal of information from implantation, but it appears that for no very good reason the results are enormously variable. A device capable of reproducing normal speech is still a long way off.

There is one interesting spin-off of this technique. Some patients undergoing the selection process for suitability for implantation are discovered to have islands of useful hearing on complex testing. These may allow them to benefit from sophisticated hearing aids giving better hearing results than is yet possible from cochlear implantation.

Cochlear implantation is established but technology is ever improving and further advances will occur. Much work still has to be done. World-wide there are many different devices being assessed and opinion is still not settled as to whether extra- or intracochlear implantation, with single or multiple channel electrodes, gives the best results. Research is also extremely expensive, not because of the cost of the devices, but in terms of time and personnel to do the complex selection, testing, and extensive multi-disciplinary rehabilitation. This is why it is only available in relatively few centres. Research will continue, but achievements often claimed in the popular press for the 'bionic ear' have to be treated with some scepticism at present. However, increased public awareness as to the problems of the deaf can only be to the good of the hearing-impaired population, and press attention does help to generate vitally needed research funds.

APPENDIX

United Kingdom

Royal National Institute for the Deaf (RNID),
105 Gower Street, London WC1E 6AH
Tel.: 01–387–8033

The British Association for the Hard of Hearing (BAHH),
7/11 Armstrong Road, London W3 7JL
Tel.: 01–743–1110

The British Deaf Association,
38 Victoria Place, Carlisle
Tel.: 0228 48844 (Voice) and 0228 28719 (Vistel)

The British Tinnitus Association,
c/o RNID (address as above)

The National Deaf Children's Society,
45 Hereford Road, London W2 5AH
Tel.: 01–229–9272

Technology Information Cenre,
4 Church Road, Birmingham B15 3TD
Tel.: 021–454–5151

Breakthrough Trust, Deaf/Hearing Integration,
Charles W. Gillett Centre, Selly Oak Colleges,
Birmingham B29 6LE
Tel.: 021–472–6447

United States of America

Alexander Graham Bell Association for the Deaf Inc. (AGBAD),
3417 Volta Place, NW, Washington DC 20007

American Speech–Language–Hearing Association (ASHA),
9030 Old Georgetown Road, Washington DC 20014

Children's Hearing, Education and Research Inc. (CHEAR),
PO Box 2000, 871 McLean Avenue, Yonkers, NY 10704

Deafness Research Foundation,
366 Madison Avenue, New York, NY 10017

International Association of Parents of the Deaf,
814 Thayer Avenue, Silver Spring, MD 20910

John Tracy Clinic,
806 West Adams Boulevard, Los Angeles, CA 90007

National Association of the Deaf (NAD),
814 Thayer Avenue, Silver Spring, MD 20910

National Theatre of the Deaf,
1860 Broadway, New York, NY 10023

American Tinnitus Association,
PO Box 5, Portland, Oregon 97207

Canada

The Canadian Association of the Deaf,
Suite 311, 271 Spadina Road, Toronto, Ontario M5R 2V3
Tel.: (416) 928–1350

The Canadian Co-ordinating Council on Deafness,
294 Albert Street, Suite 201, Ottawa, Ontario K1P 6E6
Tel.: (TTY or Voice) 1–613–232–2611

The Canadian Hearing Society (publishers of *Vibrations*),
271 Spadina Road, Toronto, Ontario M5R 2V3

The Deaf Children's Society of Ontario,
271 Spadina Road, Toronto, Ontario M5R 2V3

Voice (parent organization),
271 Spadina Road, Toronto, Ontario M5R 2V3

Australia

Better Hearing Australia,
288 Unwins Bridge Road, Sydenham 20444,
Sydney, NSW
(This organization also has branches in many other Australian
cities)

The Deaf Society of New South Wales,
PO Box 432,
Petersham, NSW 2049

Queensland Deaf Society,
34 Davidson Street,
Newmarket, Queensland 4051

Royal Tasmanian Society for the Blind and Deaf,
Argle Street,
North Hobart, Tasmania 7000

Victorian Deaf Society,
101 Wellington Street,
East Melbourne, Victoria 3002

INDEX